Am I M[illegible]usal?

Learn what to expect, [illegible]ow your body changes, and how to support it with holistic tips and tools. Journey though perimenopause with serenity.

Jo Hayns

Book Cover by Eleanor Hayns

1st edition [2023]

Contents

Preface IV

Introduction 1

1. Am I Menopausal? 3
2. Understanding Your Body 11
3. Move your Lymph 23
4. Your Hardworking Liver 37
5. Your Digestion 50
6. The World of Stress 83
7. Tackle Your Sleep 103
8. Alleviating Your Symptoms 118
9. Holistic Remedies Explained 137
10. HRT 167

What Now? 172

Interesting Reading 174

About the Author 178

Preface

For me perimenopause started when I was caring for my dying Mum, who was living on her own having lost my Dad 4 years previous. As I was the nearest off-spring living over an hour away, I went with her to all of her hospital appointments. I coped with her increasing anxiety and changing moods that occurred due to the type of cancer she was dealing with. Life was very stressful and busy. I had 2 small children, a full-on job and unbeknown to me at the time, changing hormones.

I would go several months without having a period and yet still had the symptoms like breast pain and tightness, and abdominal cramps. In addition, my skin and hair was changing, fluctuating from being dry to oily and then back to dry again.

Obviously, the time with my Mum was very stressful and emotional. However I started to second guess decisions and be unsure of whether I had made the right choices even on the everyday things I had been doing for years. I went to see my doctor who, considering my age (43) and the situation, was convinced that I was far too young for the menopause.

The reason for my symptoms was 'simply stress'. I was not convinced, so I kept going back until one day I asked for a blood test to rule it out once and for all. The results came back – probably positive for perimenopause. As you will see blood tests are often inconclusive and unreliable for diagnosing menopause. Knowing your body, trusting yourself and your observations are better.

Your experience may not be the same as mine, we are all different. Some go though perimenopause with a variety of symptoms, others are forced into it due to an illness or operation. Whatever your situation, and whether you are going down the HRT route or not, there is always something you can do to improve your symptoms and smooth your transition.

During the last 40 years as a complementary therapist I have been asked many times, 'do you think am I menopausal?'. In the early days (30 years ago) women did not know what was happening and the subject was rarely discussed. Capable women were left to fear they were losing their mind. No one prepared them for what it entailed. The research and data we have now about the menopause is mainly gathered on women who have already gone through menopause. Most of them did not use lifestyle changes to help themselves as the knowledge was not there. So, just imagine how different things will be for you when you start to help your body now!

I started doing research for this book in order to help my clients. I have more or less read every menopause book on the market. Although some of them are good at giving you information, others are extremely technical, which is interesting but not very practical. Some focus entirely on HRT, a specific diet or exercise plan and many are really depressing! This book is different.

The facts are that perimenopause is a transition, just like puberty in reverse, and your post menopause may last for 30 years or more. Given this information, I want to give my clients and now you, practical tools to sail through the chaos with serenity and age-well for longer. It is time to start planning for the next phase of your life and live it with the maximum joy, energy and health you can. This is something the women who went before you could not even dream about. They did not have the knowledge or understanding. By reading this book and implementing tips that work with your lifestyle, you will be in a better place.

Start preparing and planning now!

Introduction

As you read through this book, you will be able to pick and choose tips that resonate with you and your situation. Have a pen and paper ready to write your own plan, with dates of how and when you will incorporate them into your lifestyle. Have highlighters or whatever you use to make notes while you are reading and jot down what you will add to your daily routine, what time of day, and when you will start. There is no such thing as one size fits all. You and your life is different to the next person and your plan should reflect that. Start with one small change at a time, experimenting as you go. Remember to adapt as you change. Swap the tools that are no longer working and keep doing with the things that make you feel good.

You will see that perimenopause is not a straight line. Hormone levels (especially oestrogen) fluctuate. Sometimes the balance of your hormones will be off. Keep working on your stress levels, sleep and the other important areas featured in the chapters of this book. You may be tempted to skip to the chapter about alleviating your symptoms. However, I advise you to make sure the basics are in place first by reading the other chapters before you do that. Get to really know your own body and be honest with yourself. Solving one symptom may be a quick single fix but it will not set you up for good health long term.

You may be gradually moving through perimenopause or have been placed into menopause by an illness or operation. You may be thinking about HRT, are on it or never want to touch it. Regardless of your situation and starting point, the lifestyle changes, tips, and tools in this book will make all the difference.

Use your highlighters, notebook, favourite app, or documents on your devices to track how you are doing and the changes you are making. Writing your plan down with a date as to when you will start and what you hope to achieve, sets you up for better success. Celebrate the wins (preferably with something healthy and relaxing), rally the support of positive women and a professional (ask for help), and make tweaks where necessary. The tweaks may include checking that you are doing enough, not too much, or trying something different.

Each week write a list of what has gone well or has improved, first! Having worked with many women of all ages, I know we are very good at recalling what we have not achieved and forget to see and list the improvements that have been made. Small wins are all steps to an enjoyable, and healthy life for longer.

1

Am I Menopausal?

So you have reached a certain age, the demands of life have increased, and you feel a little different in a way you just can't quite put your finger on. You may be feeling more anxious, unable to remember names or deliberate more over the simplest decision. Are you going mad? No, you are perimenopausal and it's time to put YOU first.

Having listened to many clients going through the menopause transition, I noticed the most common complaint was increased anxiety and self-doubt. One client found the emotional changes more difficult than anything else. She was actually relieved when she found it was the menopause.

What Happens in Perimenopause?

From mid-40's onwards, the ovaries prepare for retirement by stopping egg production. The pituitary, however, not realising this is happening increases the Follicle Stimulating Hormone (FSH) and Luteinising Hormone (LH) messages, attempting to get the ovaries to mature an egg. Progesterone levels slowly decline, and oestrogen levels fluctuate. While this miss communication goes on, chaos ensues. Periods become difficult to predict. Some months you may have a very light discharge or nothing at all and then a sudden heavy period. A blood test can be an indicator, but these tests are mainly ineffective as your hormone levels change daily, hourly, or even every second. So, knowing your own body is better. These changes occur before the well-known brain fog, hot flushes, and night sweats.

As the number of hormone receptors for oestrogen and progesterone reduce, your body tries to get rid of the excess. Some of the oestrogen is stored in adipose tissue (fat cells) and these cells start to expand. The main place for this type of storage is in the abdominal and breast tissue causing an oestrogen dominance in these areas.

Added to this your life may already be stressful with elderly parents who need more attention, children or teens who need help, your work life maybe demanding leaving you less time to recharge your batteries. As the ovaries reduce oestrogen production, the fat cells and adrenals start to pick up the slack. If your adrenals are already under constant demand, they will struggle to prioritise the level of oestrogen production necessary for a smooth transition.

If you are in the perimenopausal phase due to a hysterectomy, cancer or another medical condition, your body probably has not had time to prepare itself and therefore you may need some help to slow the transition down. I suggest checking with a specialist clinic to discuss your options.

Despite how you transition through menopause, whether you opt for HRT or not, you can still make lifestyle changes to help with your symptoms and support your health.

Some women still experience symptoms post menopause and this is usually stress related. Here again you can deal with those by making lifestyle changes.

Let's pause at this point and remember, you went through puberty over time and now through menopause your body will adjust over time too. It is natural! Life will go on past the menopause for at least 20-30 years or more! It is time to prepare for this next phase and put selfcare at the top of your list.

What is Menopause?

Officially, after 12 full consecutive months of no menstrual cycles means you have reached menopause (a pause in menstruation). It is worth checking with your medical professional to make certain. Although rare, there is a chance you can still become pregnant especially if you are under 50 when this happens – better to be sure.

Post-menopause and the Rest of Your Life

When you are post-menopause, life naturally changes **but it is not over!** So, what will YOU do to enjoy the rest of your life?

Although you cannot stop menopause or the ageing process you can make changes to improve your life quality and have just as much (if not more) enjoyment than you did before. The power is with you.

What Can You Expect From Perimenopause?

Well, these are some of the symptoms that women have said they had during perimenopause. Most of them will disappear once the transition has passed. Some may remain needing further lifestyle adjustment, and/or investigation. It's not all bad! Understanding, experimenting, and taking action is key.

Some of the symptoms mask other things that have been going on for a while. The good news is that many can be sorted with better understanding, making small changes, and being kind to yourself.

Remember, hormones are one, albeit important, aspect of this next phase of your life and post-menopause your body will function differently. You do need to adjust and if like me, you are an empty nester, this may be the perfect time to re-evaluate your life. Remember what you love to do and make plans.

What Indicators do You Have?

- Brain fog
- Poor concentration
- Anxiety and panicky
- Memory lapse
- Irritability
- Mood swings

- Dizziness
- Insomnia
- Fatigue
- Headaches (or migraines)
- Hot flushes
- Night sweats
- Change in sweat and body odour
- Stress incontinence
- Muscle or joint pain and stiffness
- Vaginal dryness
- More urinary infections
- Prickly skin
- Brittle nails
- Itchy skin
- Restless leg syndrome
- Dry and thinning skin and hair
- Dry eyes
- Facial hair

- Dry or burning mouth
- Gum disease or ulcers
- Breast soreness
- Tinnitus
- Abdominal bloating
- Constipation
- Weight gain especially round the abdomen
- More food sensitivities
- Irregular heartbeat
- Palpitations
- Changes in menstrual cycle
- Low libido

Remember some of these indicators could be symptoms of something else. If you are worried or they are severe and frequent, contact your General Practitioner (Gp) to rule out any medical complications. Lifestyle changes can often be used alongside and enhance medical treatment. And in many cases the solutions are simple.

Knowledge Recap

- Menopause is a natural lead up to the liberating mid-life and beyond.

- Unless your menopause is operation or illness induced, this transition is a gradual process over time. Like puberty in reverse.

- Perimenopause can start with no symptoms at all. You will gradually feel a little different.

- There are a variety of symptoms. Those in your mix will be determined by your hormone history and life experiences, chronic stress levels, sleep, and lifestyle.

- There are many ways to help your body adjust to the new normal. Have fun experimenting.

- Understanding what is happening and why, then work out the best steps to take for you. Take action to help make your transition smoother and reduce the severity of your symptoms.

- You are post-menopause when you have not had a period for 12 consecutive months. You can be menstrual free for 6-9 months and then have a heavy bleed. This takes you back to month 1.

- If over 50 you do not need to think about contraception 1 year after your last period. If under 50, you should wait 2 years or check this out with your doctor to confirm.

- Talking to your mum (if you can) about her experience may help, but with knowledge you can make improvements.

- If on any type of hormonal contraceptive, the early symptoms will be masked. Check with your doctor to discuss the best course of action.

- If you have a bleed post menopause, see your doctor to check out why this has happened. Some herbal remedies, like red clover, may keep your menstrual cycle going longer.

Whatever your symptoms, start to plan for post-menopause. How do you want to live it? What are the things you have always wanted to do? What do you really enjoy?

2

Understanding Your Body

"You are in truth a cooperative community of approximately fifty trillion single celled citizens" Bruce H. Lipton, Ph.D., The Biology of Belief

As a community of cells, each of your citizens have a part to play and their own speciality. They all have the same DNA and genetic manual. However, each group of cells will read a different chapter from the book. All your cells are linked together and respond to their environment and each other. The wrong pH level, dehydration, chronic stress and tension, a lack of nutrients, an inefficient waste system, or not enough time for rest and repair causes them to struggle, mutate, or die.

Why is it More Important to Know About Your Amazing Body Now?

In the first part of your life, the way you can live depends on the genes you are dealt. Now, during (and post) the menopause, your continued health is down to you – how you listen to and work with your body (or whether you work against it).

So, if you feel different and cannot put your finger on why, you may question whether you are perimenopausal. You may notice your menstrual cycle becoming less regular and heavier on occasion. One of the most common symptoms women have told me about over the years is feeling more anxious, second-guessing decisions or not being able to come to a decision. If you are a businesswoman or an organiser this may be difficult and even frightening for you. Like Jackie a client of mine who said, "I thought I was going mad, until someone explained I was perimenopausal". Rest assured this is all part of the hormone chaos of perimenopause. By understanding what is happening, will reduce your stress, and enable you to get the support to reach the other side as smoothly as possible.

Some women report changes in memory, libido, weight, or feeling tired all the time. Now I see these symptoms in women before menopause too, along with restless legs and IBS type symptoms. Putting a few practical step in place can make all the difference, as you will see.

Let us first, introduce you to your body. You will then have the power and understanding to make effective changes.

"Knowledge is power; power provides information; information leads to education; education breeds wisdom, wisdom is liber-

ation. People are not liberated because of lack of knowledge."
Francis Bacon

Many of the physical solutions will have an emotional and biochemical effect too. Let's start with your hormones and the glands that run your community of cells and organs.

Your hormones and the endocrine glands that secrete them, run your body throughout your life. They have been doing this before menstruation started and will carry on long after they stop. After menopause some of the responsibilities change, like a restructuring of a company's staff. Working with the nervous system, hormones are chemical messages used to create a change or action. So, before we get down to talking about menopause solutions, you need to learn about the endocrine system. This will help understand the symptoms you experience now or may have experienced throughout your life. Some of the emotional and physical symptoms are due to the chaos of perimenopause and some will be due to lifestyle and how you deal with stress.

As I have said before, hormones are chemical messages that stick on to a cell via receptors and activate a reaction. Messages flow between two endocrine glands or an endocrine gland and a specific organ, like the heart, liver, lungs etc.

To me the endocrine glands are like the departments of a large business community. Each have a job to do, and all strive for a common aim – to keep you safe and healthy. When one department is struggling, the other departments will try to help out but over time their efficiency is impaired due to the increase in workload.

Let's now look at them in a little more detail:

Hypothalamus – *The chairwoman*

Is located on the underside of the brain just above the pituitary. Its job is to take an overview of the whole body, instigate adjustments, and maintain a steady level of function (homeostasis). Nerves bring information to the hypothalamus about internal and external changes e.g., temperature, thirst and hunger, stress, dangers, and blood pressure. Then hormones are released to instruct the pituitary to rally the other glands (departments) to act and make a change. The Hypothalamus also talks to the autonomic nervous system (ANS) and sends out messages directly to areas like bones, muscles, blood vessels etc

The hypothalamus orchestrates:

- The entire endocrine system – your hormone system
- The neurological system – nervous system
- The immune system
- Weight set point – affecting body fat changes and the weight set by your body
- The metabolism
- Heart and respiratory rate

- Temperature
- Sleep cycles
- Energy output
- Sex drive
- Fertility
- Skin colour
- Stress response or intolerance

If there is a problem with how the hypothalamus regulates these functions the following symptoms show:

- Fatigue – most common
- Insomnia
- No sex drive
- Irritability
- Depression
- Brain fog
- Changes in body fat
- Exercise intolerance
- Temperature intolerance
- Stress intolerance

Pituitary – *The Managing Director*

Is located just below the hypothalamus, underneath the brain. It oversees the daily running of the organisation from glands to organs. It orchestrates:

- The menstrual cycle
- Stress response
- Thyroid function
- Sleep
- Growth and repair
- The immune system
- Inflammation

Pineal – *The Master Timekeeper (Endocrine Clock and Calendar)*

This very important gland coordinates your senses. It is one of the biggest stores of serotonin, tryptophan and when darkness comes it secretes melatonin, your sleep hormone. The pineal also secretes the hormone responsible for starting and ending the child-bearing years. It instigates when your periods are to start in puberty and when they are to stop in menopause. The master timekeeper is the place to start if you have difficulties with sleep. Like a conductor, it sets and keeps the pace for all the organ clocks working together.

Thyroid – *The Metabolic Regulator*

Located in the front of the neck in the shape of a butterfly. This gland regulates the heart rate, metabolism, muscles, digestion, brain development and bone maintenance. In times of constant stress, it has been known to helps the adrenals when they become too tired to function.

Pancreas – *The Blood Sugar Controller*

Located by the stomach and small intestine. This gland has dual purpose. The endocrine part secretes hormones to control blood sugar levels, while the digestive part produces enzymes to digest protein, fats, and carbohydrates. When blood sugar rises the pancreas secretes insulin to allow the muscles, liver, and fat cells to take the glucose to use as energy. When blood sugar is too low, the pancreas secretes glucagon to convert stored glucose in the liver and fat cells to be released back to the blood stream.

Parathyroids – *The Calcium Controllers*

Small glands located behind the thyroid. Calcium is tightly controlled in the blood. When low, parathormone signals to the bones to release calcium and to the kidneys to stop getting rid of calcium in the urine. Parathyroids activate vitamin D to increase the absorption of calcium from food in the gut. One of the reasons why your Vitamin D levels are so important.

Adrenals – *The Stress Responders and Sex Developers*

Located on top of the kidneys, they each have an inner part called the medulla and outer part called the cortex. The medulla is responsible for instigating the physical responses to stress. It will prepare the muscles, affect heart rate, breathing, energy supply and increased alertness for fight or flight. The cortex is responsible for making testosterone, oestrogens, progesterone, and cortisol from cholesterol.

Ovaries – *The Production Department*

Ovaries produce oestrogen and progesterone to affect the development of an egg and the lining of the womb. If an egg is not fertilised the balance of oestrogen and progesterone initiate menstruation.

The Heart – *The Supreme Conductor and Figurehead*

More than just a pump, this little organ commands and synchronises the rhythms of the body. It tunes in and listens to the composition of the blood and sends messages via nerves and hormones to regulate and balance the body. As an endocrine gland it lowers blood pressure by instructing the adjustment of salt levels and affecting blood pressure hormones, produces neurotransmitters like dopamine, and noradrenaline, and has receptors for many other hormones including oestrogen. The heart constantly communicates with the brain and the gut.

Adipose tissue – *The Energy Stores*

In women, this tissue tends to be around buttocks and thighs. You also have a thicker layer under the skin than men. The distribution of these cells change with age when oestrogen production changes. Adipose tissue stores excess energy and releases it when necessary. The hormones of adipose tissue help regulate glucose, cholesterol, and steroid hormones (oestrogen, progesterone, testosterone, cortisol etc)

There are other systems in your body that are worth a mention here, as they are important services for your efficient body at any age.

Support services:

Lymphatic – *The Waste Service*

This forgotten system needs attention. Cell waste is transported though lymphatic vessels to nodes. These are like recycling depo's that filter out useable and repairable items, neutralises foreign bodies and separates the waste. Only when the lymph system clears cell waste can fresh nutrients feed the cells. It is more important to get this system working right than concentrating on your diet. For this it relies on muscle contraction, effective breathing, and massage to move the fluid through your body. It is also a big part of your immune system.

Digestion – *Fuel and more*

In my time as a therapist and kinesiologist tracing the root causes of client's issues, I always end up somewhere in the digestion. You can eat a wonderfully healthy diet but if you cannot extract those nutrients they end up down the toilet. Equally, if you cannot get rid of waste efficiently your liver and cells suffer. Digestion and urinary systems work together to get rid of waste. Your gut bacteria plays an amazing part too.

Liver – *The Toxic Waste Processor*

Your liver is rich with blood vessels, nutrients, and needs plenty of energy to process the toxins. Fat soluble waste like micro-organisms, contaminants and pollutants, food additives, medication and alcohol are processed by the liver to make them water soluble. Then, all water-soluble waste is eliminated either through the kidneys and bladder in the form of urine or mixed with bile in the solid waste and out. Some of your symptoms through perimenopause are signs that your liver is struggling under the pressure of extra work from the increase of excess oestrogen to process. So, being kind to your liver and taking the pressure off as we age is a smart thing to do.

Blood Circulation – *The Transport Network*

Moves hormone messages and nutrients like oxygen around the body to where they are needed.

Muscular and Skeletal – *The Structure and Movement Maintenance Department*

This is not just about movement, but your bones and muscles help with energy supply, creating new red blood cells and supply of nutrients like calcium. As seen above this department is vital for moving fluid around the body via the lymph system and thereby helping the immune system too.

Kidneys – *The Fluid Controllers*

Essential for regulating the level of water, and minerals (like sodium, potassium, and calcium) in the blood. Kidneys are involved in the removal of liquid waste, and excess water, which in turn regulates the blood pressure. They activate vitamin D for strong bones and when oxygen in the blood is low, they produce a hormone that stimulates bone marrow to produce more red blood cells to increase the oxygen levels.

Brain – *The Personal Assistant*

A complex part of the nervous system, who's functions are too numerous to mention. Your brain is a main player in holding and attempting to make sense of the messages from your environment (outside and inside). It also files away experiences and pulls out information when needed. 4 of the senses are only contained in the brain and the other 2 are all over your body. Although, you may consider your brain to only be in your head, in fact, in recent years there has been growing evidence that your head's brain talks to your heart brain and your gut brain. Also, there are more messages sent from your heart (which reacts fast to the environment) to the brain and the gut than the other way round.

Knowledge Recap

- Although there are many departments within your body, they all work to a common goal – to keep you safe and healthy.
- Keeping active, breathing effectively, sleeping well, and eating a balance diet, is more important now, than ever before in your life.
- Sort out your weakest area and the rest will be able to work more efficiently. This is usually the neglected lymphatic system, your liver, and your sleep.
- Take control of your stress, be kind to your liver, work that lymph, and think self-care.

3

Move your Lymph

You have to remove the waste before your cells can take in nutrients!

The main jobs of your lymphatic system are to remove cellular waste, supervise and inform the immune system, and fat absorption. If your lymph flow is polluted, clogged or stagnant, your cells are compromised. When cells are living in a toxic environment, they become full of inflammation and unable to get the oxygen and nutrients they need.

This system touches every other system and cell type in your body, which is why we are starting here. Over the years I have so often found that my midlife clients are eating well, exercising and still they feel tired, unwell, and cannot lose weight. Lymphatics are the key. Clearing out the waste means that your cells can feed!

Like the blood circulation, the lymphatic system has a network of tubes all over your body. These vary in size and follow the same routes as blood vessel and nerves. The primary function of the lymph system is to run the waste collection service, picking up fluid filled with waste from the around every cell and take it to nodes. The nodes filter out invaders and remove harmful substances. They destroy and take away worn-out cells so they can be replaced with new ones.

Lymphatic vessels have very low pressure with only valves to make sure the fluid goes in one direction. All the fluid from around the body makes its way to the subclavian veins under the collarbones. Here it is put back into the blood stream.

The Thymus is made of lymphatic tissue and its main function is to promote the development and maturing of T-lymphocytes (T-cells) which fight foreign organisms that may infect your body. From infancy to puberty the thymus gland is large as it learns to enhance the T-cell range and then it starts to shrink. Your thymus produces hormone-like proteins to help mature and differentiate T-cells. As far as we know the hormones of the thymus are involved in the immune response. The thymus and its hormones also influence other organs and systems including kidneys, spleen, reproductive system, and central nervous system.

The spleen is often described as being about the size of a small fist. It has a rich blood supply that brings T-cells from the thymus, B-cells from bone marrow and macrophages. These are all used as part of your immune response to invaders. The spleen filters your blood and stores red blood cells and platelets. It will become overwhelmed if the lymphatic system has blockages. The spleen and liver work closely together.

Nodules of lymphatic tissue are positioned in places where there is mucous membrane and where invaders can enter your body. This includes the digestive, urinary, and reproductive tracts, and your respiratory airways.

Tonsils found at the back of your throat, Peyer's patches found in your small intestine and your appendix at the end of your caecum (a pouch where your small and large intestine meet) are made of lymphatic tissue.

Your digestion and brain are linked. Any issues with the digestion affects brain function, which in turn affects the digestion. This happens via cranial nerve 10 called the Vagus nerve. We now know this important wandering nerve affects the heartbeat, all abdominal organs, controls inflammation, and decreases the stress response.

Your lymphatic system is important for managing the waste from your cells and tissues, moving the fluid around the body, controlling inflammation and is a big part of your immune system too. In complementary therapy treatments, it is said if there is nothing else work on, always work the lymphatics.

During Perimenopause

With lower oestrogen levels, lymphatic and blood vessels, will lose elasticity and become stiffer. Over time this makes the job of both these systems difficult and less efficient.

As your hormones fluctuate, the lymph circulation, and detox mechanisms especially the liver have an extra workload. Working your lymph system (and helping your liver) is key to helping the body be more efficient.

As a kinesiologist and reflexologist, I work on the lymphatic system to improve the whole body and to stimulate blocked areas where fluid has become stagnant. Some of these techniques you can do at home with great success and your will see many of them through out this book.

The best ways to move fluid through the lymph system is:

To breathe well. The mechanism of breathing, draws the fluid from extremities to the centre of the body and up to the larger lymph vessels.

To move. If you sit or stand still for any lengths of time you may have found your ankle swell at the end of the day. Keep moving your feet, ankles, and toes. Set your alarm every half an hour to get up and move around (or maybe get some more water). If you are on a call and can be mobile pace up and down the room. This is not only good for your step count but brilliant for your lymphatic system too. Regularly do the **calf pump** (see below) and stand on one leg while cleaning your teeth or waiting for the kettle to boil. These all help with the sensitivity of your feet and balance as you age.

When the lymphatic system has become stagnant in places, you need to rub specific points. See the map in this and the other chapters for specific rubbing points. Each spot relates to a muscle, a meridian and specific organs too. However, when you rub an area which is tender, keep rubbing for up to a minute and then stop. Continue rubbing the following days for up to a minute until the tenderness is no longer there. Always start at the collarbone and centre of the body and work out.

Any form of **massage** or **reflexology** techniques work the lymph system very well. There are also specific massage techniques like Reflexology Lymph Drainage (RLD) or Manual Lymph Drainage (MLD)

Knowledge Recap

- Your body cannot work effectively unless it clears out the cellular waste first.
- Working the lymph not only improves the quality of life for your cells and tissue, but also improve your circulation, nerves, digestion and urinary too.
- Start working your pelvic floor, as you will be using those abdominal organs and clearing waste, a lot!
- Start slowly, and if in doubt contact a health professional, especially if you have medical complications.

Essential Oils

See Chapter 9 to check for cautions with individual oils, especially if you have medical conditions

Basil, sweet - cleansing

Chamomile, German – anti-inflammatory

Cypress – diuretic and decongestant, stimulates the liver and pancreas, and balances excesses.

Eucalyptus globulus – cooling and decongesting

Fennel, sweet – strong diuretic

Frankincense – aids deep and slow breathing

Geranium – waste and congestion remover

Hyssop – anti-inflammatory and decongestant

Marjoram, sweet - diuretic

Melissa (Lemon balm) – calming and anti-inflammatory to all tissues.

Niaouli – tissue toner

Oregano – diuretic, may increase sweating so use sparingly and experiment.

Palmarosa – hormone harmoniser and fluid retention balancer

Peppermint – cooling, decongesting, and anti-inflammatory

Ravensara – stimulating for aches and pains.

Rose otto – strengthening for lymph vessels.

Rosemary – circulatory tonic, clearing fluid retention.

Sandalwood – astringent and decongestant to circulation.

Thyme – anti-inflammatory

Reflexes

Hand

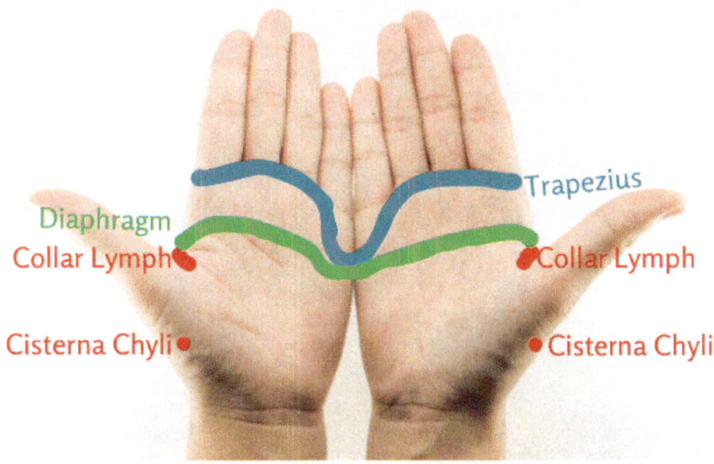

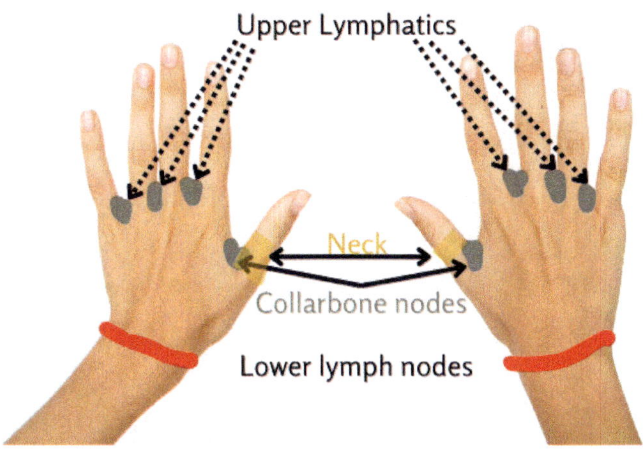

Ear

Rub these points. If any feel sharp, keep rubbing. (See Chapter 9 for more information on working reflex points)

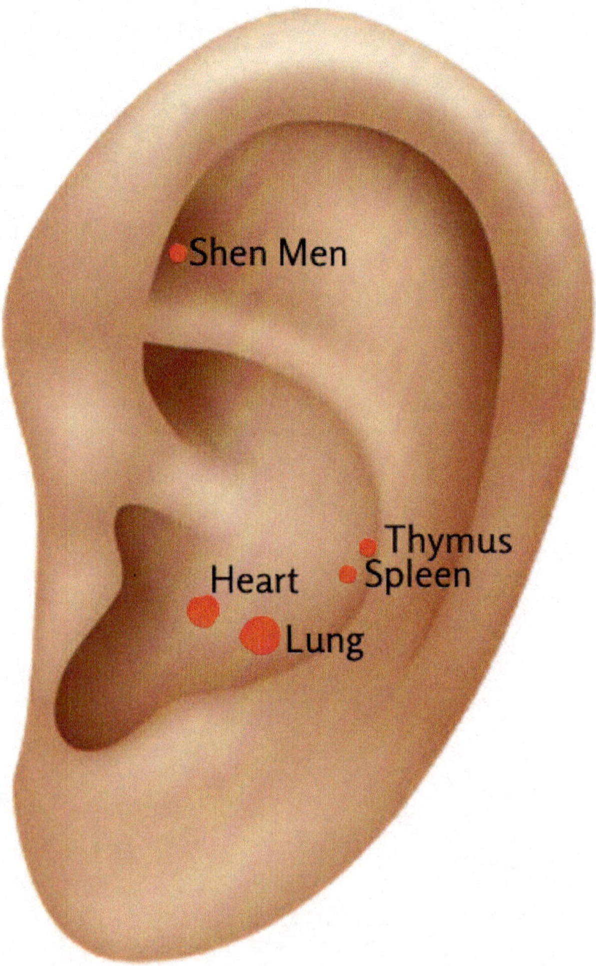

Face Yoga Routine

Rub and tap in this order:

- Above and below the collarbone
- Under the earlobes
- Under the jaw
- The cheek area just in front of the ears
- Nasal folds
- Temples (and into the hair above and behind the ears)
- Back of the head from ear to centre
- From the armpit around the shoulder to the collarbone.

For visual instructions, go to YouTube and explore the videos on my channel @serenitymojo7134

Rubbing Points

These are effective when rubbed, tapped, or gently thumped with a loose fist but whatever you do work them lightly and experiment between vigorous, slow or or a combination of both to each point. It is important for lymph techniques that your do them in the order shown in this list:

1. Above and below the collarbone

2. Sternum – down the centre, and either side where the ribs attach
3. Vagal points – the soft area behind the earlobe at the back of the jaw
4. Axillary – from the outer edge of the collarbone to the armpit.
5. Around the navel
6. Inguinal – in the crease of your upper leg from the pubic bone out
7. Behind the knee – work just above and below the crease
8. Jump up and down (the calf pump explained below is the safest option especially if you have knee pain, or a large chest!)

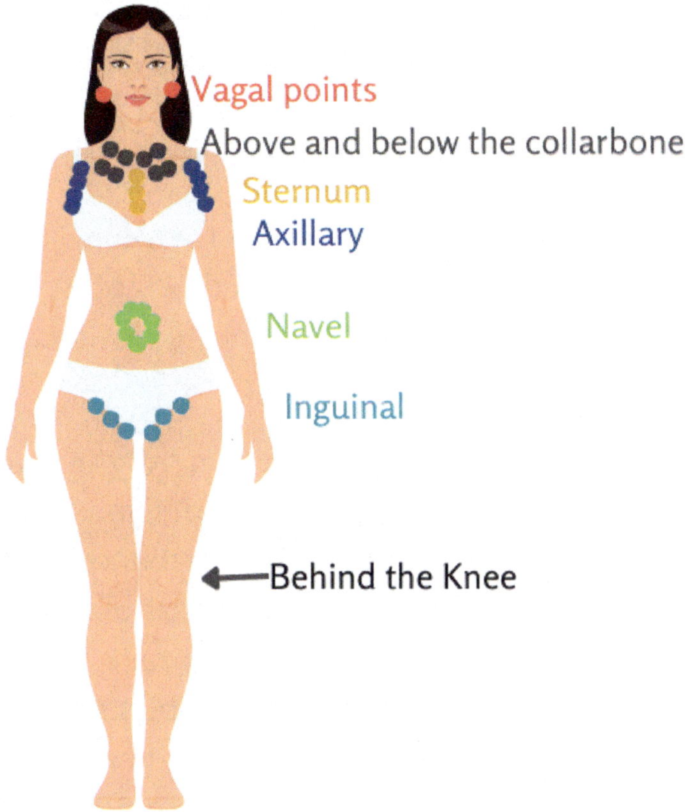

Movement

All movement is good for the lymph system, but key movements that most people forget are:

Spinal twists – either seated in a chair or on the floor or lying on the floor. You will find many examples on YouTube. Start slowly if you are new to these exercises as they seem simple but can be very challenging.

Salutations to the sun – is great for waking up the body and moving every joint. Choose a version you are comfortable doing.

Leg lift – spend time lying on your back with your feet up the wall. This can be restorative to the brain and heart. You could move your legs to exercise them and encourage fluid to return to the centre of the body.

Calf pump – while standing with arms and knees soft, bounce by lifting both heels up and down off the ground, keeping the balls of you feet and toes in contact with the floor.

Foot exercises – moving your feet is very important to your general health and especially to work your lymph back up to the main vessels under your collarbone. Exercises to strengthen and tone the tendons and fascia of your feet also connects the peripheral nerves to your brain. This is crucial as we age. It prevents falls, and aids foot stability, spatial awareness, and foot issues like arthritis, hammer toes, although go gently with these. The way the body is constructed means that all the different parts of your body are connected by special tissue called fascia. This has to be kept hydrated, strong, and flexible. Fascial tissue that is compromised in one area creates tension in other places and also impairs how nerves work, organ efficiency, as well as waste disposal and blood supply.

Foot exercises include:

- Moving them under your desk
- Pacing while on a call
- Standing on one leg in turn while cleaning your teeth

or waiting for the kettle to boil

or you could go further and do some specific exercises like these:

1. From seated or standing, place your feet flat on the floor, raise your heels on to the balls of your feet and press down to stretch the ligaments under the foot. Roll back to the heels and raise your toes (or just raise your toes if standing).

2. Stand with your weight equally in the middle of 3 points – under the ball of your big toe, under your little toe, and middle of your heel. If you are not sure whether you are balanced between these point rock your feet to the outsides, here your knees should move outwards and thighs rotate in your hips too. Now rock to the inner edges of your feet, moving your knees towards each other, and thighs rotated inwards. Then place your feet flat and rock your weight forward and back. Feel for the middle of these points.

3. From the position above lift all your toes up off the floor and spread them out before placing them on the floor. From there scrunch the tips of your toes by pressing the tips into the ground. Try concentrating on one foot at a time at first. Hold for about 5-10 seconds and then relax, repeating 5 – 10 times for each foot. As you do this you will feel the arch of your foot increase and the ball of your foot lift slightly off the floor. Practice this every day but if it hurts of

tightens in the beginning give yourself a rest day in between.

Alternatives and additions:

- Place a towel on the floor and try to move it by scrunching it up.
- Press big toes down into the floor and lift the other toes up
- Press big toes and little toes down into the floor and lift the middle three toes.

Breathing

Place linked hands on your lower ribs with little fingers just above the navel.

Breath normally, in and out through your nose.

Then, as you inhale notice your hands moving out and relaxing as you exhale.

Each time you inhale, push the ribs and abdomen outwards.

Focus on the sides of the ribs for a couple of breaths.

Then in the next couple of breaths, focus on the back of the ribs.

Continue for a few more breaths applying a little pressure with the hands each time you breath out and relaxing the hands as you breath in. Repeat this 5-7 times

4

Your Hardworking Liver

Known as the General or Chief of Staff in Traditional Chinese Medicine (TCM). The word liver in old English is Lifer

Your liver is a hard-working organ situated on the right side of your upper abdomen and just under the diaphragm. Most women are unaware they have a liver issue. Muscles associated with the liver are Pectoralis Major Sternal (across the chest) and Rhomboids (between the spine and inner edge of the shoulder blade). If these muscles are tense and tight, your liver (and lymphatic system) may be struggling.

Other indications your liver is stressed are panic attacks and angry outbursts, or irritability at others or yourself. Physically, you may be aware of your heart pounding, or you may become less tolerant to alcohol. If you are in mid-life and developing an increase of weigh around the belly and you have been told that your cholesterol and blood pressure is creeping higher help your liver work better.

The liver is responsible for filtering, detoxifying, nourishing, replenishing, and storing blood. It stores a large amount of sugar in the form of glycogen that can be released into the blood as glucose when energy is required. The liver receives amino acids from the small intestine, which it changes into different forms for the growth and repair of body tissues.

One main job of the liver is to recognise harmful toxins and help detoxify them from your body. It does this in 2 phases:

Phase 1 – the waste is modified and put out for collection, like bagging up your household rubbish ready for the dustbin cart. This phase works quickly and is able to speed up when there is more waste to modify.

Phase 2 – the waste is changed from fat soluble to water soluble. The waste can then be eliminated from your body through the kidneys in urine or in bile wrapped up in stools (usually in fibre!). Different toxins need different substances to process them.

If you imagine the liver as a large recycling plant, you can understand that if there is too much waste coming in problems will start. Phase 1 processing will speed up while phase 2 struggles to keep up. The result in this case, is the incoming toxins have to be stored back in body tissues.

A good blood flow is necessary for the liver to function. Also, the liver makes bile which is then stored in the gall bladder. By the age of 55 (brady 2015) bile production is reduced by 25%. So, with much to do and a tiring liver the bile becomes too concentrated. Breaking down fat and animal protein (containing fat) is difficult, and stones are common. Bile lubricates the intestines and stimulates peristalsis (the contraction of intestinal muscles that push the stools through the tubing) resulting in hard dry stools that accumulate in the small intestine causing constipation.

From a TCM perspective, the liver controls the peripheral nervous system regulating muscular activity and tension. An inability to relax is often a liver meridian dysfunction. Liver energy controls ligaments, tendons, and muscles, it regulates movement and physical coordination. So, ***relaxation is key.***

During Perimenopause

In your youth, your 20's and 30's, the liver can process anything you send it. Your ability to eat and drink what you like is down to the genes you inherited at birth. Now in your 40's, perimenopause and beyond, your liver's efficiency is under your control. Why is this? Well, your liver has been working hard for many years and is now tiring. As stated before, your liver needs plenty of blood to function. Lower oestrogen affects the flexibility of your blood vessels. This can mean that blood pressure and cholesterol levels can increase along with belly fat. Due to the bile issue explained above, the risk of gall stones and constipation is higher.

As the number of oestrogen and progesterone receptors decrease there becomes an excess of oestrogen needing to be processed by the liver. If your liver cannot process it all, the excess will end up in fat cells. So, menopause adds to the liver's workload.

Knowledge Recap

The liver is hardworking and can easily become overwhelmed in the chaos of menopause – be kind to it during this time. It is not all about reducing or cutting out alcohol, although that will help! The good news is that you liver constantly renews itself and can heal in 6-8 weeks of making changes. Here are some things you can do:

- Remove foods that are causing you bloating in your small intestine. These tend to be wheat based but for you it may be milk, processed meat, or other foods that you are eating constantly. If you are not sure what these foods are write a food diary of everything you eat and drink for a week. Your sensitivities are usually the one thing that you eat every day. Remember that one woman's nourishment is another woman's poison! So, ignore what you read in the press or what you friends say, your sensitivities may be different. Equally there may be another reason for your bloating! Visit a kinesiologist to test or see a nutritionist.

- You may be eating the same type of food for breakfast, lunch, and dinner. For example, you may be having toast for breakfast, a sandwich at lunch and pasta in the evening. Experiment with changing your bread to sour dough or forget the bread and have pasta instead. Pasta is denser than bread which makes it slower to digest and chew, making it less likely for you to overeat.

- Follow a mainly alkaline diet full of vegetables, that have plenty of vitamins like vitamin C, water (to reduce retention) and fibre.

- Eat less in one sitting. You could use smaller plates and chew slowly. Get used to leaving food on your plate when you are full.

- Remember your liver, brain, and muscles love the glucose. Eat whole foods like brown rice, oats, and fruit in the morning. Water full foods like cucumber, celery, tomatoes, soups are also great.

- Keep processed and fatty meat, dairy, fried foods, and snacks to a minimum.

- Use vinegar, water, broth, wine, or dry fry as a method of cooking or succumb to an air fryer, (it's not just for frying).

- Choose organic, fresh, or frozen whole fruits and vegetables wherever possible.

- In short, avoid the chemicals in processed foods and drinks including sodas, juices, and smoothies. Instead, juice and smoothy your own. Eat whole, unprocessed foods mainly from plants, often the ones without nutritional labels.

- To reduce inflammation and also increase flavour, add herbs to your food. Best for the liver are dill, caraway seeds, rosemary, sage, thyme, ginger, garlic, and turmeric. Ones that are roots or bulbs, like ginger and garlic, can pick up chemicals from the ground. These can be good and bad, so buy the best quality or organic if you can.

- Some people like to use lemon juice in water first thing in the morning to flush out the liver. Drinking this in the morning and then exercising seems to give the liver a boost of energy. Remember to rinse your mouth with plain water afterwards to avoid weakening your tooth enamel. Another idea is to use good quality vinegars (like apple cider, red wine, balsamic etc) over your salads, soups, vegetables, bread etc.

- Drink tea like green, chamomile, ginger, peppermint, or Caraway seed, if tea is your thing.

- Remove all the things that are not serving you well from your cupboards. Out of eyesight and out of reach is out of mind. Start by detoxing your kitchen and throw them away. Instead, fill your cupboards with healthy nutritious foods that fill you up with essential nutrients. These are naturally colourful foods.

- Start to look at the labels. If something in the shop has a nutrition label showing the amount of fat, sugar, and salt it has been processed already.

Essential Oils

See Chapter 9 to check for cautions with individual oils, especially if you have medical conditions. All essential oils and especially ones that are high in Ketones, can build up in the liver. To avoid this, use with care and change the oils in your blend monthly.

Black pepper – stimulates the liver and a sluggish digestion.

Camomile, Moroccan – bile stimulator helping a congested liver and colon.

Cypress – stimulates liver secretions.

Eucalyptus dives - aids liver function

Ginger – warming stimulant

Grapefruit – for sluggish liver problems, right-and side discomfort, and slow burning issues.

Juniper berry or twigs – stimulates secretions.

Lemon – helps with the acidity in the body.

Mandarin – helps breakdown fats and is calming to the digestion.

Neroli – liver tonic

Orange, bitter – liver stimulant

Orange, sweet – calming and a tonic.

Peppermint - cooling decongestant

Rose otto – cleansing for the liver.

Rosemary - tonic and stimulant

Reflexes

Hands

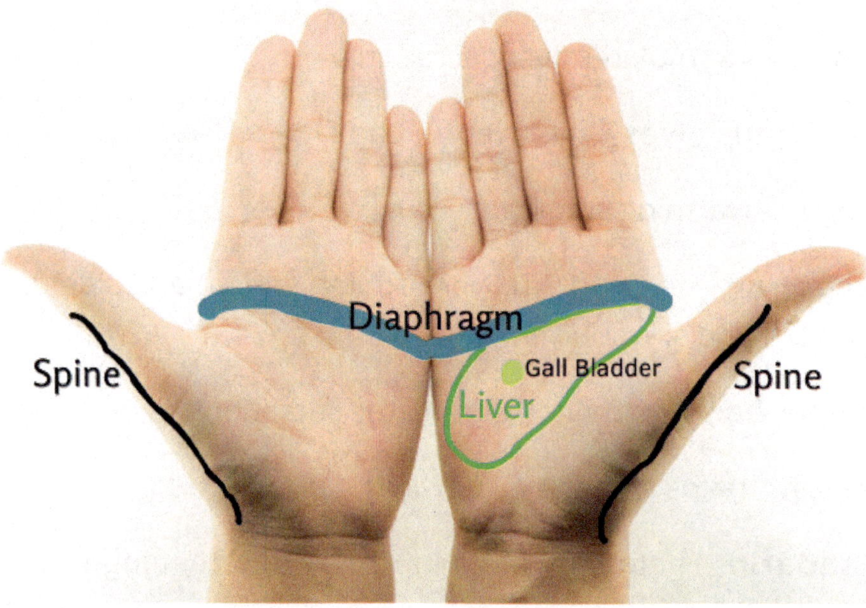

Ears

Ting Zhong – abdominal pain and bloating

Temple – for pounding, throbbing, and one-sided, around the eye, temple, or side of the head that occurs when the gallbladder, liver, and digestion needs stimulating.

Liver, Gall Bladder, and Liver yang

Shen Men – supports the other reflex points

Rub these points. If any feel sharp, keep rubbing. (See Chapter 9 for more information on working reflex points)

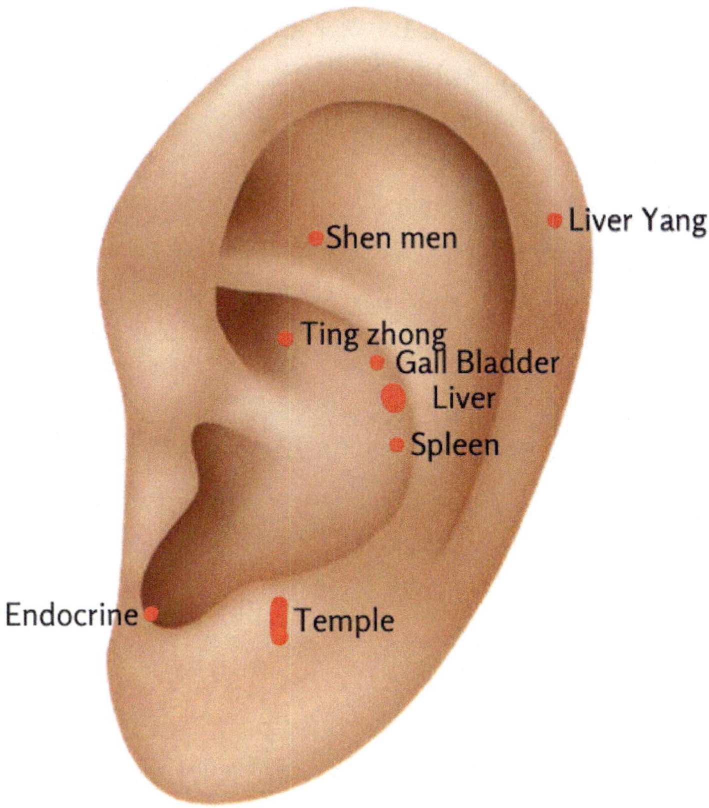

Face Yoga Routine

- For the liver rub up and down over the area between

eyebrows at the root of the nose

- For Gallbladder rub beside the eyes at temples
- Rub Point 0 right in front of the ears by stroking up and down.
- Hold the glabellar point found between and slightly above the eyebrows for 40 secs. This balances the master glands.
- Press on the Adrenal points found over the roots of you canine (pointed teeth) for about 40 secs. Notice if either side is feels different
- Hold the ESR points (seen below). You can locate these with the thumb and finger of one hand. They are in line with the pupils of your eyes when looking forward and half way between your eyebrows and hairline. Alternatively, place one hand over the forehead to connect these points.

For visual instructions, go to YouTube and explore the videos on my channel @serenitymojo7134

Rubbing Points

For the Gall bladder – lightly and quickly rub the crease behind the knee, and hold the soft spot on top of your head.

Rub between ribs 3-5 and 5-6

Rub over GB31, you can find this point by standing with arms relaxing down the side seams of your jeans or trousers. where the end of the middle finger touches on that seam is this pressure point. If you are unsure rub up the outside seam. If there is a problem it will feel tender.

For the Liver – hold above Emotional Stress Release points (ESR) located on the forehead. These are between your eyebrows and hairline, in line with the pupils or your eyes. Hold these points using the thumb and finger of one hand. Alternatively you could place one hand over your forehead. There needs to be a connection between the 2 points to aid general relaxation and help the liver too.

Rub between ribs 5-6 on right side only

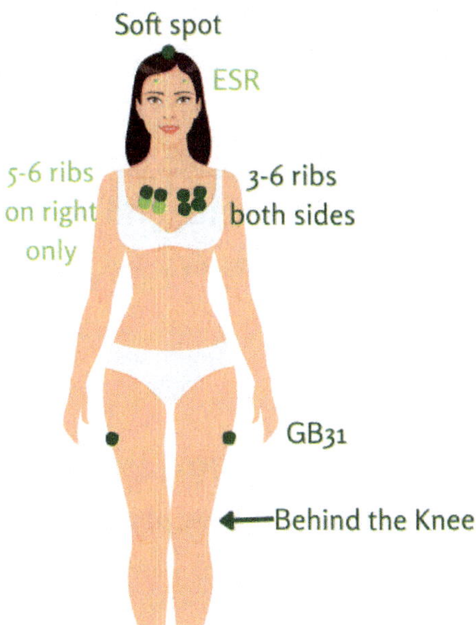

Movement

Backward stretches can be as simple as sitting on a chair or the floor, pulling up out of your hips with shoulders relaxed and with a little tension between the shoulder blades. Make sure the back of your neck is lengthened and chin is slightly down. Now lean back, opening up your chest towards the ceiling or sky. If you are supple you can progress on to more challenging back stretches over an exercise ball or yoga block. Start gently and keep within your own body's capability. These stretches should be relaxing and held to allow gravity to work its magic.

Spinal twists are always good for massaging the abdominal organs. You can do these seated, lying on the floor, or standing. Choose a position that suits you where you can move in a relaxed way. Go slowly focusing on each part of the spine. This is a movement that we forget to do in everyday life and yet it is a movement that should be part of our routine. If your spine is stiff don't over do it. You could simply stand, soften your knees, relax you arms, and gently twist using the momentum of your arms as you rotate from side to side.

Breathing

Sit with lips are gently closed, and tongue rested or pressed to the roof of the mouth. Exhale fully to prepare

Inhale for 2 seconds and hold your breath for 2 seconds, holding your diaphragm steady. Then keep repeating the inhale and pause until your lungs are fully inhaled. Depending on your lung capacity this may take 4, or more times.

Exhale deeply and slowly through your nose, gradually relaxing the diaphragm.

Repeat 8-10 times

Practice a few times daily, like morning and evening on an empty stomach.

5

Your Digestion

Your digestion is truly amazing and the key to your continuing health.

It is heavily influence by your emotions, stress levels, your circadian rhythms, sleep quality, the diversity of your microbiome, and yes, your hormones!

While going through peri menopause, there is a decline in oestrogen throughout your body. This affects the brain, heart, breast tissue, liver, digestion, uterus, bones, blood vessels, muscles, and joints. As oestrogen (and progesterone) decreases cortisol rises and adrenaline may be triggered too.

What Does This Mean for Your Digestion?

More stress hormones (adrenaline and cortisol) switches on the stress response and switches off the digestion. You may find there is a sudden bowel evacuation or digestion stops causing constipation. Many women comment that they have IBS type symptoms.

High cortisol will reduce stomach acid levels, keeping the food in the stomach for longer and slowing the transition time of your digestion. Enzyme levels that work on digesting your food reduce too. Therefore, making you more prone to bloating and discomfort as the food is not digested efficiently.

Gut tissue changes and becomes more sensitive and inflamed. Some of the bloating and constipation can be caused simply by the loss of elasticity in the gut which is slowing the system down.

All is not lost keep reading!

How Does Digestion Work?

Your digestion gets to work when you smell and see a delicious plate of food. This can be part emotional and part survival instinct.

We can put that to the test:

Close your eyes now and imagine the smell of your favourite dish wafting into the room. In an instant, part of your brain remembers when you experienced that smell before. Memories flood your brain with the place where ate it, the friends you were with, the joy (or pain) you felt, but more of that later.

While you remember the experience, another part of your brain is analysing the food. Is it a danger or pleasure, do you need to activate the troops to kill invaders or produce the right enzymes to work on what is about to enter your body?

You take a bite

There is a rush of saliva, made up of water and all-important enzymes, ready to sterilize and cleanse the mouth and get to work breaking down the food.

There is an explosion of taste flooding your brain with memories again. Ah! you know what this is, you have eaten it before, it's a combination of protein, fat, and carbohydrates. As well as the sending messages to your brain, some go to your stomach, shouting "get ready food is on its way".

But there is one more thing you need to do, and this is the part most people belittle and think is unimportant.

The chewing!

A full workout involving teeth to grind up the food into smaller pieces and a tongue to moves the food around and bashes it on to the gums. Not only does this heighten the taste and experience but it stimulates the saliva glands to produce a glut of enzymes. The more work done here, the more efficient the job done further down, and the less energy that is needed.

Now your bite of food, wrapped in mucous is swallowed down and moved along a tube by a wave of muscle contraction. In fact, it takes about 6-8 seconds to reach the stomach.

So far, the environment has been slightly acidic and this is about to ramp up. The stomach contracts every 20 seconds, churning your ball of food, mixing it up with gastric juices. Previous work on the carbohydrates mainly ceases now. The stomach acid takes over, destroying unfriendly bacteria in the food. Here a mixture of acid and enzymes start to break down the bonds of the proteins, stretching out the curly protein bonds.

Depending on the food you have eaten, your stress levels and your personal transition speed, the churned-up food passes out of the hectic stomach into the small intestine after about 4-6 hours.

Now in the small intestine your food is ready for the absorption stage. Linked to the first part of the small intestine are the pancreas and gall bladder. These secrete two enzymes: those from the pancreas work on undigested protein, the fat, and the rest of the carbohydrate. The gall bladder expertly squirts out bile to emulsify fat enabling it to be digested.

Bile also stimulates the circular muscles found along the 6-7m of intestine, in order to push your food mix through slowly. All the way along mucous protects and lubricates the tubing, while hair like structures and a more varied set of enzymes break down your now liquid food into tiny particles that can be absorbed. This is the 'good stuff' that is taken off to the liver to be sorted, processed, and sent wherever it is needed.

Your liver works hard, and its health is so important that is has its own chapter. So, if you skipped that part go back and give it a read at some point.

By the end of the small intestine all that is left is undigested food and fibre. Your gut cannot digest this type of fibre. It is there to be worked on by your gut microbes as it carries on its journey into the large intestine. Feeding these helps your health as they secrete waste that is made up of essential nutrients for you and help to liberate vital minerals.

Between the large and small intestines is a valve called the ileocecal valve (ICV) which opens to allow digested food to pass through and then shuts to stop this waste from returning back. Sometimes, this valve can become too relaxed, too tight, or too sensitive (when it opens and shuts randomly). You can tone this valve and help it to work efficiently by seeking advice from a Systematic Kinesiologist, or Chiropractor who specialises in ICV treatment. When your skeletal muscles and/or connective tissues are tense, this can affect the ICV too.

Now, hopefully, all the nourishing parts of your food have been absorbed. What is left is squeezed round the large intestine allowing your gut bacteria to feast and ferment. Gas is removed and if some undigested protein has slipped through, nitrogen can cause an unpleasant smell. Slowly the water content is taken out and the bulk is passed out.

Knowledge Recap

Throughout this chapter I have mentioned your gut bacteria. By this I mean your gut microbiome, which is in fact made up of different forms of bacteria, yeasts/fungi, viruses and other organisms. To make things easier we will collectively call them bacteria. For it to work harmoniously for you, the gut microbiome has to be carefully balanced.

High stress affects the way you digest. A nerve called the Vagal nerve wanders from your head out to the organs of your body. Anxious thoughts, shock, nervousness, trauma, and excitement affect the stomach and intestines. You may have experienced this and said, “I feel sick to my stomach” or “I feel like I have butterflies in my tummy”.

During and after menopause when oestrogen and progesterone production is lower can cause:

- The sensitivity of your gut lining to increase leading to leaky gut, inflammation, food sensitivities
- Higher inflammation levels throughout your body, as it mostly starts in your digestion.
- A change in rate of food transition, making it slower causing a higher chance of constipation.
- Bowel elasticity to reduce causing more bloating.
- Secretions like stomach acid and enzymes to decrease.

- A lack of diversity with your gut bacteria
- Your appetite to change
- Your serotonin levels to lower

The following symptoms show your digestion needs some attention:

- Dark circles under the eyes
- Catarrh and sinus congestion
- General achiness or itchiness
- Headaches
- Joint pain or stiffness that cannot be stretched out and where no other treatment has fixed it
- Body or breath odour
- Fluid retention
- Constipation and/or diarrhoea
- Bloating, reflux, wind, or burping
- Memory impairment
- Feelings of disbelief and misunderstanding
- Feeling detached or indifferent.
- Feeling of apathy or despair.

- Tinnitus, ringing, or whistling in the ears (this can also be due to an infection, poor lymphatic function or nerve impingement)
- Chronic fatigue especially where you completely shut down.
- Fatigue and lethargy
- Less forgiving
- Dizziness

What Can You Do?

Eat Healthy Foods

Going back to the basic principles of eating whole foods that have not been processed, with plenty of good fibre (fruit, veg and legumes) and a moderate amount of fat and protein.

Avoid foods that have nutrition labels and where nutrients have been added as these will be over processed, manufactured and lacking the good stuff.

Your Microbiome and Fibre

You have more bacteria cells than human cells and most of that bacteria live throughout the gut. In fact, it is a rich and diverse ecosystem. Why do we allow and even encourage this? Simple, because they repay your hospitality by balancing your hormones, digesting your food, boosting your immune system, and making available vitamins and other chemicals that are useful for your mood and vital to your health.

Keeping your bacteria happy and healthy should be one of your top priorities! What you eat affects the type and diversity of your bacteria colony and subsequently your health and weight.

Fibrous whole foods feed your gut bacteria, and also strengthen the muscles and integrity of your intestine. These fibrous foods come from vegetables, fruits, nuts, seeds, and legumes. They contain great nutrients to support you through the rest of your life.

It's not you that digests the fibre but your bacteria which thrive on it. In return they reward you with vitamins like K, and chemicals like short chain fatty acids (SCFA).

SCFA help:

- To indicate to your brain, you are full and stop you from overeating.
- Help regulate blood sugar levels
- May help in weight loss
- Reduces inflammation and block cholesterol production
- Protect the lining of your gut

More positive research is coming out all the time. There is one note of caution before you start to increase your fibre intake. If you have inflammatory bowel conditions, wind and bloating increase the fibrous foods slowly. Remember, it is your gut bacteria that digests this food and you need to change the quantity and diversity of that bacteria in order to be effective at digesting the fibre. Too much too soon may make symptoms worse. Your gut bacteria changes very quickly but you may need to allow your digestive tract time to adjust. Nevertheless, adding fibre to your diet is like a healthy workout for your digestion. Like any training programme you would not for example run a marathon on day one!

So called 'Good" bacteria, works with your body and rewards you. In contrast, "bad" bacteria do not work with you and in large numbers can cause more bloating, diarrhoea, inflammatory bowel diseases, diabetes, obesity, liver diseases, heart conditions, cancers, more food intolerances and generally make you feel unwell.

You will not eliminate the bad bacteria; it is about creating a balance and having more good bacteria than bad.

Make sure your valves are working

If the ICV is open for too long, closed for too long or open and shuts randomly, waste matter can be absorbed back into the body without going through the normal processes. A compromised ICV can produce all sorts of symptoms inside the gut as well as fatigue, poor concentration and unwanted emotions, skin sensitivity and disorders, itchiness, joint and muscle aches and pains.

The Houston valves are the 2-4 c-shaped rings at the top of the rectum that control the exit of solid waste and help to support the weight as it accumulates. This valve is like a chicane in a road that slows the traffic down. A compromised Houston valve always has an emotional element attached (anxiety or stressful situation) and will result in constipation and/or diarrhoea.

Often symptoms are random, varied and do not seem to link together. These are the women who come to my therapy room. Chiropractors and kinesiologists will physically fix these valves. Kinesiologists will also look at the associated emotions, nutrients, foods, and sensitivities etc.

The Histamine Effect

I see many women who have suffered from digestive aches and pains, itchy scalp, tiredness in the form of a complete shut down and yet have no medical issues. This may not have been an issue before but during the menopause chaos you may notice this more. I suffered from a histamine issue during my perimenopause years with constant sneezing, itchy head, panic feeling and extreme tiredness. With a few adjustments to my diet and lifestyle this is no longer a problem.

Histamine is a natural chemical called a neurotransmitter and is a messenger used by nerve cells when they talk to each other. It is sent to instigate your immune and inflammatory response. It also plays a role in the function of your gut (where most inflammation begins). Its primary job is to get rid of allergens.

When histamine is released it causes a slight irritation. The inflammation alerts the body that an invader is present. This signals the white blood cells showing them where to find the invader and causes blood vessels to swell so more white blood cells can arrive to attack the invader. Once the invader has been dealt with, the natural response is for enzymes to break down the histamine to prevent a build-up and any problems from occurring.

When histamine is not broken down, an intolerance can develop. Some medications can increase your histamine levels and some foods either contain or increase histamine levels. When levels are high, the body is under stress causing an allergic type of response. An intolerance can accumulate, producing symptoms when levels are pushed over the edge making identifying a single cause tricky to identify.

Symptoms of this include:

- Irritability, depression, anxiety, brain fog, vertigo/dizziness
- A rash, flushing, hives
- Joint pain
- Racing heart, palpitations, hypertension, arrhythmia
- Altered bowel function, abdominal pain, nausea,

vomiting, abdominal cramps, non-celiac gluten sensitivity, reflux/GERD/heartburn

- Nasal congestion, runny nose, sneezing, difficulty breathing
- Insomnia, fatigue
- Headache, migraines
- Abnormal menstrual cycle
- Tissue swelling

Reducing stress levels, cutting out fermented foods, improving your sleep quality, checking your thyroid, and avoiding your known irritants will all help. Changing high impact exercise for lower-impact, using weights and stretching before bed can reduce stress and subsequently histamine levels.

If a histamine intolerance is your issue, here are some of the foods and drinks to either cut out or cut down:

Vegetables

Eat

Fresh vegetables including:
Fresh Fennel
Artichoke
Asparagus
Beetroot
Bell Peppers
Bok choy
Broccoli
Brussels sprouts
Carrots
Cauliflower
Celery
Collard greens
Courgette
Cucumber
Garlic
Green beans
Kale
Leeks
Lettuce
Onions – red and brown
Parsnips
Sweet potatoes
Swiss chard
Turnips
Watercress

Nibble

Mushrooms
Peas
Pumpkin
Squash

Avoid

Aubergine
Spinach
Cabbage
Sauerkraut
and other fermented vegetables
Prickly pear
Stinging nettle
Milk Thistle

Fruit

Eat

Fresh or frozen
Apples
Apricots
Blackberries
Blueberries
Cherries
Exotic fruits
Figs
Grapes
Pears

Nibble

Raspberries
Kiwi
Lemon
Lime
Mango
Nectarine
Papaya Peach
Plum

Avoid

Citrus fruits
Avocados
Bananas
Pineapple
Strawberries
Tomatoes
Melon
Dried fruit:
apricots
prunes
dates
figs
raisins

Starch & Flour

Eat

Gluten-free grains, bread, and pasta
Brown rice
Quinoa
Coconut flour
Tapioca
Oats

Nibble

Almond flour

Avoid

Soured breads
Wheat germ
Couscous
Wheat

Legumes

Eat

Avoid for a few weeks and then reintroduce some carefully

Avoid

Bean's
Lentils
Peanuts
Soybeans

Nuts & Seeds

Eat

Macadamia
Pumpkin seeds
Chestnuts

Nibble

Soaked almonds
Pecans
Pistachio
Soaked Brazil
Pine nuts
Flax seed
Sesame
Sunflower
Pumpkin

Avoid

Walnuts
Peanuts
Cashews

Animal Protein

Eat

Freshly or frozen
Chicken
Turkey
Duck
Lamb
Pork
Beef
Fresh fish:
Salmon
Sardines
Free-range Eggs

Avoid

Left overs
Cured meats:
Bacon
Salami
Ham
Pepperoni
Hot dogs
Shellfish:
Crab
Lobster
Oyster
Shrimp
Canned fish:
Tuna
Smoked fish:
Mackerel
Anchovies
Sardines
Fish sauce

Fats

Eat

Extra virgin Olive oil
Coconut oil
Organic Ghee
Grass-fed butter

Dairy & alternatives

Eat	Nibble	Avoid
Coconut milk	Mozzarella	**Fermented dairy:**
Rice milk	Ricotta	yogurt and kefir
Hemp milk	Cottage cheese	**Soured dairy:**
Almond milk	Cream cheese	cream, milk, buttermilk
Raw cow's milk		Aged cheese including goat
		Cow's milk

Drinks

Eat

Herbal teas
Water
Peppermint tea
Pomegranate juice

Avoid

Wine especially red
Champagne
Beer
Kombucha
Kefir
Alcohol in general
Energy drinks
Coffee
Black and green tea

Other

Eat

Leafy herbs
Celtic or Himalayan
Sea salt
Black Pepper
Ginger
Peppermint
Thyme

Nibble

Apple cider vinegar
Dried herbs and spices

Avoid

Fermented soy
Soy sauce
Miso
Vinegar
Pickles
Mayonnaise
Olives
Artificial preservatives
Dyes
Yeast

Intolerances and Balance

As I said before, one woman's food is another woman's poison. We are all as individual as your combination of bacterial species. You can change your microbiome quite quickly by eating different foods. If you have checked your valves and reduced your histamine levels and still have intolerances, here is what you do.

Intolerances can be to any food. So, using a journal can give you extremely useful information. Write down what you eat and when, your symptoms (emotional or physical) and when they occur . You can do this for many of the menopausal symptoms like hot flushes, concentration and brain fog, joint aches, and pains. What you are looking for are patterns like when I eat bread, I feel sluggish and the top of my head itches.

Remember, it can take a while for food to move throughout your digestive tract so the timing of symptoms may not match exactly to the timing of foods eaten. However, keep going and you will identify the patterns. If you eat the same foods daily or many times a week, they are more likely to cause issues. **Variety is key!**

Some foods and products can be grouped together as they contain the same naturally occurring chemicals that do not work with your gut. For example: atropine is found in tomatoes, potatoes, aubergine, bell peppers, chilli's, egg, and tobacco. If the foods you sensitive to seem random, it may be a chemical that links them. That chemical may also be in your home, workplace, or personal care products too.

Kinesiology testing for these is the quickest way of identifying your triggers.

Some intolerances occur when you have a shock, trauma, or major emotional event. When this occurs, your body remembers what you are doing and what you are digesting. This can create an emotional link between the event and the food in your stomach at the time. If you have had an intolerance to a particular food, go back to when it started and ask yourself what happened around that time.

Leaky gut

When your skin becomes very dry and cracks, the protective barrier is not complete and allows bacteria in, creating sores. In the same way, your gut lining can become weakened and cracks can appear. This allows bacteria to slip through, triggering an immune response and ultimately inflammation. On your skin, the acid mantle (a mixture skin oils, amino acids from sweat and the skin's microbiome) creates a barrier to protect it from invaders. In your gut, specialised cells form a barrier by producing a mucus layer and this acts as food for your bacteria when they do not have fibre to feed on. Your gut also has its own lymphoid tissue which irradicates the invaders, but these can be overwhelmed if your lymph system is overstretched, and your gut lining is leaky.

Raw fruit and vegetables not only feed your bacteria but introduce bacteria to your gut too. With raw foods it is even more important to chew, than cooked food. Before you go and buy probiotic supplements, it is now thought that feeding your bacteria is better for repopulating the supply than adding to it. Try this first and then consider a short course of probiotics. As I have said before, it takes less than a week to change the biodiversity in your gut. That means eat more plants! They have been producing protecting substances for a long time. Plants produce of all kinds have bacteria and eating a variety is key. Always wash your fruit and vegetables and if possible, eat some raw. In general, you will find the good bacteria on the inside of the plant matter, not the outside.

Your gut biome is unique to you and is influenced by the things you eat. There are 2 main species and a few extra ones that researchers know of so far. These are:

Bifidobacterium – usually beneficial and generally found in the large intestine as they are anaerobic which means they live without oxygen. This group of bacteria love foods containing inulin like garlic, onions, and Jerusalem Artichokes. Polyphenols also help to increase this group of bacteria species. Eating berries, most fruits, and vegetables such as apples, pears, and peppers, and having drinks like, green tea, and coffee (without milk as this blocks the benefits)

Lactobacillus – are found in the small intestine as they like to live in an aerobic environment. Foods that stimulate the growth of these are generally the fermented foods like kefir, kombucha, sauerkraut, and also cottage cheese, miso, and tempeh.

A prebiotic is the food feeds your gut bacteria. Just like any pet, your bacteria needs you to make sure they have a constant supply of water, the right environment, and the right type of food.

Simply put this means fibrous tissue from fruits, vegetables, herbs, spices, legumes, nuts, and seeds. Eat a variety over the week and if you are new to eating these in large quantities, build it up slowly.

Intuitive eating

This is beneficial when you have lost the ability to notice when you are full, or you eat mindlessly or for emotional reasons before realising you are making poor choices for your body. Include the use of a journal to help you identify food, emotions and symptoms that link together.

Eating mindfully starts with gratitude. When presented with your plate of food connect to feelings of gratitude for what you see, like the farmers who grew it, the drivers who transported it etc.

Then take time to see the colours on your plate and notice the textures by sight and if you can by feel. Smell the food and imagine what it will taste like.

Only now take a bite and focus on the texture. How crisp or mushy it feels in your mouth and the actual taste. Allow the food time in your mouth to chew before swallowing and then repeat the whole process again.

Doing this for at least one meal a day not only helps build a better relationship with your food and the enjoyment of eating but will improve your digestion and the nutrients absorbed leading to more energy and better mood.

Knowledge Recap

- Eating is memorable – if with friends and good times it is a pleasure (be mindful of portion control)
- Eating with sadness, stress, chaos, or trauma can create sensitivities and problems for your digestion.
- Remember that you are either in fight and flight mode or rest and digest mode. Relax when eating to give your body the best chance at using your food for maximum benefit.
- Chewing is a very important part of removing all the goodness out of the food (chewing and using your tongue helps eating and swallowing as we age and remedies against breathing difficulties, clogged sinuses, and snoring!)
- Eat mindfully to slow things down, notice when you are full, and develop a better relationship with your food. Use the intuitive eating routine once a day.
- Make sure your digestion is working well. Profession-

als to consult are a Systematic Kinesiologist, Chiropractor, or Osteopath who specialise in posture and digestion.

- Eat the best quality food, packed with the most nutrients and taste. These are the raw ingredients that feed your body and mind.

- Eat plenty of raw or cooked vegetables, some fruit, and legumes to feed your friendly bacteria to keep you healthy, full of energy and balanced with nutrients.

- Eat whole foods with plenty of fibre to give your digestion a workout and improve the muscle contractions making it strong, fast, and regular.

- Eat food that contain water to aid your food transition and hydration.

- Take a break from eating by fasting overnight to allow your digestion to recover and clean itself. If you aim to stop eating by 8pm this will help you to maintain your blood sugar levels easier. Insulin is tolerated better in the mornings when your body expects you to be active and less tolerated in the evening when it assumes it is bedtime. This will affect how you cope with sugary foods, simple carbohydrates, and proteins too. Only eat fruit in the morning

Essential Oils

See Chapter 9 to check for cautions with individual oils, especially if you have medical conditions and sign up for a course on how to blend oils at home here

Anti-inflammatory – Benzoin and Bergamot

Balancing blood sugars – Benzoin, Eucalyptus, blue gum

Digestive calming – German Chamomile, Frankincense, Lemon, Lime, Mandarin, Marjoram sweet, Melissa (Lemon balm), Bitter orange, Neroli, Petitgrain, Patchouli, Sandalwood

Stimulant – Black Pepper, Cinnamon leaf, Clove bud, Eucalyptus blue gum, Geranium, Ginger, Juniper berry, Ravensara, Rosemary

Warming – Ginger

Antiseptic & antiviral – Coriander, Tea tree, Thyme Common, Sweet

For bacterial infection – Coriander, Sweet fennel

For expelling parasites – Bergamot, Chamomile maroc, sweet fennel, Thyme common red or white

Fungal reduction – Myrrh, Sweet orange

Reflexes

Hands

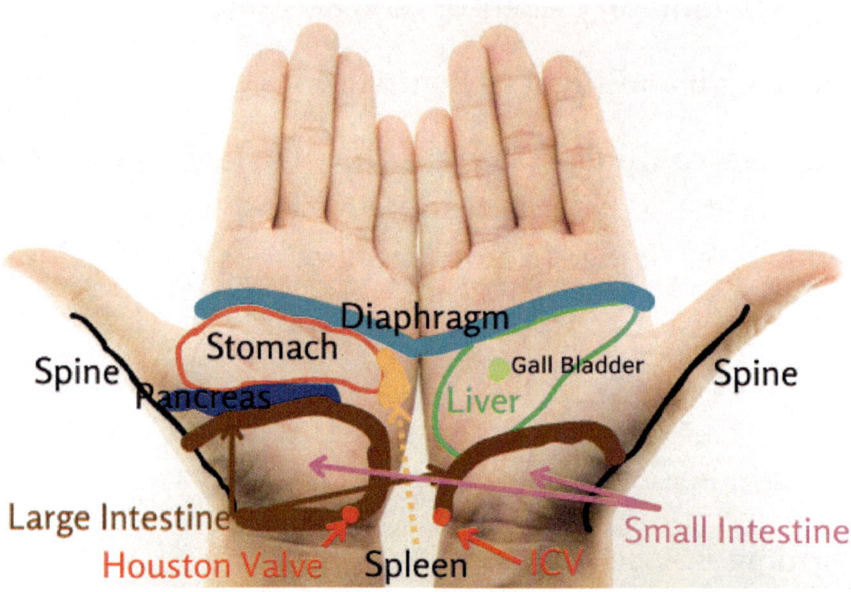

Do not worry too much about the positioning of the points. Rub the palms as indicated with your fingers, a wooden tool or the blunt end of a pen. Any tender areas, work gently to stimulate the reflexes, reminding the body where there is work to be done.

Ear

Rub these points. If any feel sharp, keep rubbing. (See Chapter 9 for more information on working reflex points)

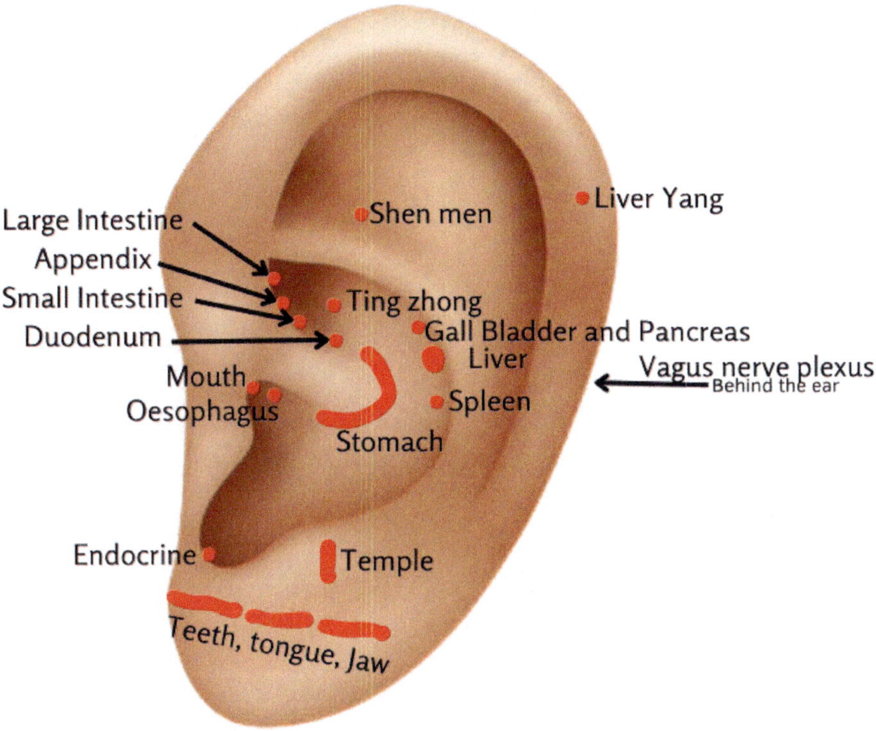

Face Yoga Routine

The best routines to work the digestion are loosening your jaw, working the plexus areas on the face, especially the solar plexus. You will find visual instructions and face yoga classes on YouTube. Explore the videos on my channel @serenity-mojo7134

Rubbing Points

Stomach – between 5-6 ribs on left, inner and outer collar-bone

Spleen and pancreas – between 7-8 ribs on left

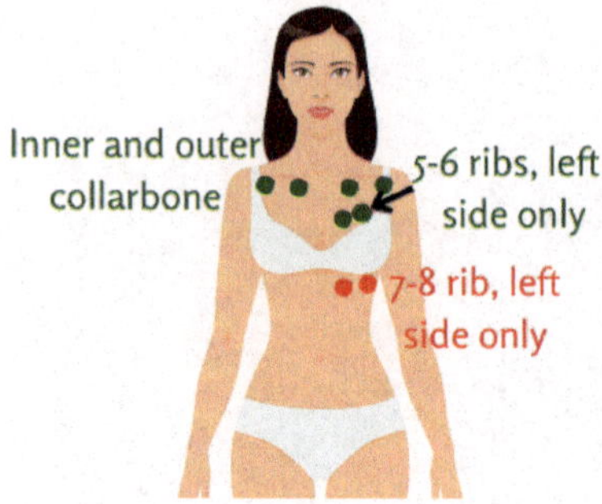

Large intestine – Tensor Fascia Lata (TFL) – outer thigh, inner thigh, and Anterior Superior Iliac Crest (ASIC) – front upper hipbone

Small intestine – between 2-3 ribs, lower edge of rib cage, inner thigh

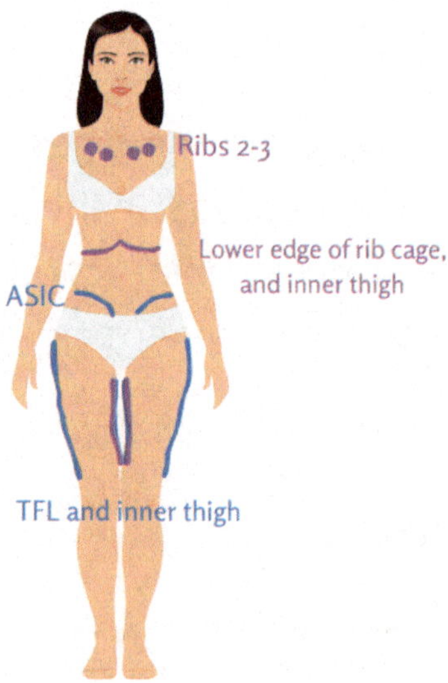

Brain and diaphragm – around the shoulders

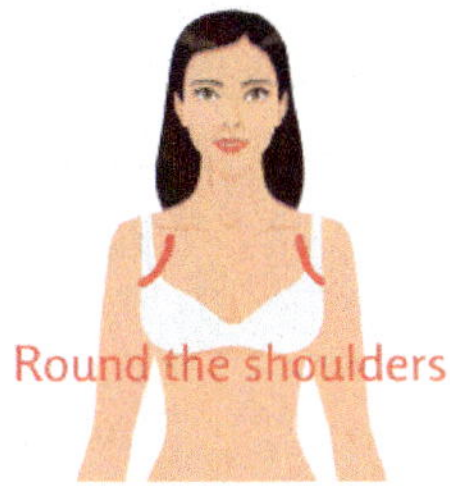

Movement

Spinal twists as explained in the previous Liver chapter are great for the all digestive organs and tract.

The bridge exercise either pushing up from the floor or over an exercise ball gives the digestion a stretch. Roll down movement is great to counter the previous bridge posture.

You could look up how to do a bow pose where you lay on the floor face down and lift up head, shoulders, and feet, stretching back with the hands to hold the ankles. If this is too strong for you, lift up the legs and upper body separately, holding for a while.

Another good digestion exercise is the lions pose. This involves slowly and steadily constricting every muscle in your face and body as you inhale. To do this you pull your arms in, crossing them over at the chest with hands in a fist. Curve your back forward and pull an angry face with eyebrows frowning and eyes tightly closed. Then as you exhale, slowly and steadily expand your arms out arching back with a roar or "ha" to relax all facial muscles, sicking out your tongue, and widening eyes to a stare. Repeat many times. This is a great coordinated movement that is not only good for the digestion but is also great to expel stress, and waken your face. Maybe do this one in private as you may frighten co-workers! Although you could get them involved in practicing it with you.

Breathing

Solar Plexus

Start by simply focusing on breathing in and out through your nose. This is always good to practice.

As you breath, check that your jaw is relaxed, shoulders are comfortable, and the back of your neck is lengthened.

Now, take your attention to the solar plexus located behind your navel.

Inhale allowing the abdomen and rib cage to expand, exhale engaging the abdominal muscles and pulling your navel toward your spine. Make this one fluid movement, where you inhale fully and then exhale fully without stopping.

Practice for 5 breaths in one session, increasing to 18 or so as it becomes easier.

Digestion breathing

Sit or lie in a comfortable place. If it helps place one hand on your abdomen around your navel. Focus on the movement this hand as you breathe.

Inhale through your nose and feel your abdomen expand. Hold your breath for 2 seconds and then exhale slow and steady.

If stressed the out breath can be through your mouth. Make it longer than the in breath and keep the mouth relaxed.

Repeat for 5 minutes to start and work up to 15 mins over time.

Bellows breath

Sit comfortably.

Prepare by taking 3 deep breaths, expanding your ribcage completely with each breath

To begin your lips can be sealed. Inhale deeply through your nose with a quick, forceful breath, and exhale the same way forcing the air out of your lungs. repeat a few times.

Inhale as before letting your chest expand and ribs open. This should be a big, strong, quick, and full breath followed immediately by a quick full exhalation.

Try to keep your shoulders, face, cheeks, and mouth muscles relaxed.

Inhale and exhale forcefully in quick succession in, out, in, out each with a full breath.

The inhalation and exhalation should be equal strength and approximately the same duration. Do not worry if the sound is loud.

If you become dizzy, stop.

When starting this techniques take a full breath (in and out) every second. Do this about 5-8 times then breathe normally and repeat after a minute. As you get confident with this increase the speed, number of rounds, and how many you do.

6

The World of Stress

Stress – "the nonspecific response of the body to any demand for change."
Hans Selye (1936)

The definition above explains that stress is simply a reaction to **anything** requiring the body to make some changes to keep it in a state of balance. The state it strives for is homeostasis (a balanced state your body aims for to keep you alive, safe and well). Homeostasis is achieved by, for example, regulating body temperature, stabilising blood pressure, or controlling blood sugar levels. Your body is doing this all the time, even now!

Through his research, Hans Selye identified that when your body comes across a stressor is goes through 3 stages:

1. ***Alarm*** – where your body releases hormones in preparation to fight the stressor or flee from it.

2. ***Resistance*** – adaptions are made to cope with the stressor and at the same time keep your body functioning.

3. ***Exhaustion*** – when resources are depleted, and your

body can no longer cope having the stressor around. This is when disease creeps in.

Stressors can be physical or emotional demands, and their threat can be real, perceived or subjective.

Stress gets a bad press but some of it is good for you! For example:

In the sleep chapter you will read about cortisol (a stress hormone), which gets you out of bed and going in the morning. This is your body saying 'move and find me nutrients'. Short burst of stress like this is called acute stress and the response soon passes.

Chronic stress is longer acting and lasts over a long period of time, giving you less time to come down from the burst of energy. Stressors that trigger this response may be one continuous thing like work pressures, constantly connected to different screens or there may be multiple things that accumulate like this:

You leave the house having had a disagreement with your partner or kids. On the way to work you get stuck in a traffic jam and are going to be late for your meeting. On arrival, you get an email of another job that needs doing and at the same moment a parent phones you. There is an emergency, and they need your help now!

Chronic stress seems never ending. Just one thing after another and even the thought of life makes you stressed!

Every time the stress response is triggered your body enters the alarm stage. As a result, your blood pressure and heart rate increases, bronchioles in your lungs dilate, muscle tension is increased, and your liver starts converting stored sugar to glucose. Digestion decreases, as this takes vital energy to process the food and extract the nutrients. Nausea, vomiting, and diarrhoea is not uncommon. Your body makes a call to stop producing reproductive hormones as who wants to bring a new life into the world when there is danger? All this is great if you need to fight or run away but your body must relax and get back to normality.

Whether the danger is real, imagined, threatening, or a challenge, your brain starts the HPA axis sequence of events. HPA stands for the hypothalamus pituitary adrenal axis as these three hormonal glands often chat and work together. The hypothalamus picks up on a threat, fear, or stressor usually from the nervous system and brain. These may be perceived as the brain interprets information gathered from the senses. Being the chairwoman, the hypothalamus converts these messages into a hormone memo and sends it to the pituitary. In turn the pituitary signals to the adrenals to release cortisol and adrenaline into the blood. The response is all the physical effects seen in the paragraph above.

During Perimenopause

Chronic stress at any age is damaging, leading to extreme tiredness, increased risks of diabetes, obesity and other metabolic disorders, depression, and reduced immune system. In perimenopause, chaos reigns, oestrogen is fluctuating, progesterone is reducing, placing even more stress on your body as it tries to work out the new norm. More stress speeds up the hormone decline, and worsens the menopause symptoms like hot flushes, night sweats, mood swings, and sleep disruption. This leads to more stress and so it goes on in a big interwoven loop. Not only that, as your ovaries have decided to retire, the adrenals now have the job of producing most of your oestrogen. They produce this weaker form of oestrogen from the same ingredients that make cortisol and adrenaline. So, if they are producing stress hormones, they are unable to produce the amount of oestrogen necessary.

This means, if you do nothing else, reducing your stress levels during menopause and incorporating plenty of selfcare is an absolute healthy priority.

Factors affected by the HPA axis:

Sleep – As cortisol levels affect sleep quality. Don't worry the sleep chapter is next, where you will tackle your bedtime routine.

Food – some foods you eat will help to calm while others will increase the stress response. Avoid the simple carbohydrates, sugars, and highly processed foods as this causes inflammation and puts extra stress on your body. Cut out any foods that do not agree with you.

Eating food after 8pm puts extra stress on controlling insulin levels.

Eating too much meat late in the evenings can stress the digestion making your body feel tired. Then you wake up in the night as it struggles to digest the food.

Eating foods that help your gut bacteria is a great way to go.

Foods that help:

Complex carbs - grains, beans, peas, lentils, and starchy veggies

Omega 3 fatty acids - fish oil, salmon, sardines, anchovies

Potassium - avocado, leafy greens, tomato

Prebiotic rich foods - onions, garlic, leeks, asparagus, apples, bananas

Probiotic fermented foods, yoghurt, kefir, sauerkraut, kimchi

Vitamin C - citrus fruit and berries

Your Jaw

Part of the HPA stress loop. The jaw is the hip joint of your head. Often, if your hip girdle (pelvis) is out of balance the jaw is affected and vice versa. The pelvis affects the vertebra of your spine which pulls on the shoulders. The temporo-mandibular joints (TMJ) is located in front of your ears and connects your lower jaw to the temporal bone above and behind the ear. Between these bones is a disc, like the ones found between your spinal bones. The TMJ are the most influential joints in the body. 50% of the sensory and motor nerves are devoted to the TMJ. Due to its location the muscles that work this joint are involved with chewing, talking, yawning, and swallowing. It also has an effect on the ears and many cranial nerves that run close by.

When stress is detected by the hypothalamus, whether that is dietary, physical, emotional, or external, muscles throughout the body tense up. This includes those around the TMJ, as well as the muscles of the heart, digestion etc. As the jaw is clenched tight, the dental distress call is sent back to the hypothalamus which tightens the jaw further.

During perimenopause, when the hypothalamus and the rest of the management team are struggling, this cycle happens more frequently. Therefore, some of the menopause symptoms, like teeth problems, gum issues, ear conditions like tinnitus, and headaches can be treated by relaxing the jaw and associated muscles.

Your Ultradian Rhythm

In the next chapter on sleep, you will learn about your circadian rhythm that runs over a 24 hour period (or actually 24 hours and 11ish minutes!). However, your ultradian rhythm is the biological cycle your brain moves through over the day. These cycles have peaks when your brain's activity is optimal and troughs where it may be sluggish, operating at a lower activity level. At peak times, blood circulation increases which causes an increase in appetite, arousal, and brain function. In the trough times, your brain takes a breather in order to recover from intense activity. These cycles occur many times through out the day. Researchers suggest that the peaks of activity can be maintained for around 90-minutes, before entering a trough of around 20 minutes.

Knowing this can help you to plan your day and work with your brain a little better. The trough period may be a good time for some breathing exercises, relaxation, mindfulness, or meditation.

Knowledge Recap

- The HPA axis creates the stress response which affects many functions of the body including hormone production that is declining during menopause.

- In perimenopause, the job of producing oestrogen falls to the adrenals (and fat cells). If they are busy making stress hormones, they are not making steroid hormones.

- Given that all the hormone glands including the hypothalamus, pituitary, and the adrenals in the HPA axis are affected during menopause it is easy to enter a stress loop that increases your symptoms.

- The stress loop can carry on into post menopause if not addressed. If your hot flushes, mood swings etc are still happening post menopause, check with your doctor, and/or combat your stress levels.

- The jaw is part of this stress loop and is an easy way to reduce stress levels or stop it getting out of hand. It also has a big influence on all muscles, nerves including the cranial ones, ligaments, and joints especially in and around the hip.

What Can You Do?

Reduce your toxic load

Some chemicals or mixes of chemicals are known to interfere with your hormone system. Some mimic hormones and others block your natural hormones. These disruptors put added stress on your hormone messengers and give extra work for your lymphatic system and liver too. Looking at your toxic load and reducing it can be very beneficial physically and emotionally.

Hormone disrupting chemicals can be found in your food, your personal care products, and household items as well as cleaning products and your local environment. You can find out more about this on the websites in the interesting reading section and by searching for good apps that you can use as you go about your day.

Mindfulness Meditation – there is now a lot of evidence that practicing regular meditation regulates cortisol in just a few weeks. Now before you say you don't have time for that, or you hate sitting still, there are many ways to meditate that does not involve sitting cross legged staring at a candle! Meditating is not about clearing your mind as that is impossible. Here are some pointers:

- 2-5 minutes of mindfulness when you wake or as you are going to bed is better than 20 minutes once a week or when you remember.

- To meditate, find somewhere that is quietish, with no distraction, and where you will not be disturbed.

- Some days it is easy, and other days even 1 minute is almost impossible. Every day is a new day.

- Aim on noticing sounds, thoughts, smells etc. and watch them all pass you by like the clouds, without reacting.

- There are many brilliant apps you can use. One of my favourites is Headspace especially if you are new to meditating and want to learn more about it. Calm is also quite good for guided sessions and relaxing music. For guided meditation, I think it is important that you like the voice. So you may have to try a few until you find what is right for you. If you look on my YouTube channel @SerenityMojo you will find some free meditations there.

- Doing some form of art. You could choose pottery, drawing, painting, or colouring. Anything that gives your mind a rest in a calm way is great.

- Qigong or Tai Chi are practices that combine slow movement, with breathing that induce a mediative state.

- Dancing, walking, even jogging.

- Listening to music. The best for relaxation and calming the nervous system are baroque, instrumental, or binaural music. If you have Spotify there is a Serenity playlist by Jo with the type of relaxation music I play in my therapy room.

Other tips include:

- Take breaks from work. Remember your brain works intensely for about 90 mins and then takes a break to recover.

- Incorporate time for yourself, take a bath, read a book, put on a face mask.

- Address any sleep issues, see the next chapter.

- Keep hydrated.

- Eat more foods containing vitamin E and Omega 3

- Reduce your caffeine and alcohol intake.

Essential Oils

See Chapter 9 to check for cautions with individual oils, especially if you have medical conditions.

Bergamot – balances the hypothalamus, for agitation, fear, stress, and anxiety.

Cedarwood – sedative

Clary sage – for sedating, panic attacks, obsessional thoughts, and regulation of serotonin and dopamine

Jasmine – restores confidence, is calming and hormone like

Lavender, true – for anxiety, irritability, headaches, stress, and sleep problems

Lemon – good for the HPA axis

Lemongrass – for nervous exhaustion, cutting through mental clutter and concentration.

Melissa (lemon balm) – a cheery oil for reducing anxiety, nervousness, and when feeling overwhelmed.

Orange, bitter (citrus aurantium) – good for the HPA axis, clears the mind and lifts the emotions.

Patchouli – for stress, anxiety, helping the mind to be more objective.

Petitgrain – for stress related conditions and nervous exhaustion to relieve irritability and promote sleep.

Rosemary (Rosmarinus officinalis) – to balance the adrenal cortex. For over tiredness, tension, and fatigue to lift the spirits and stimulate the mind.

Sage (Salvia officinalis) – to balance adrenals

Thyme common, sweet – when feeling fatigue and to balance the adrenal cortex.

Ylang ylang – for when you are feeling overwhelmed, over sensitive, stressed, tense and mentally exhausted. This deeply relaxing oil will help to sedate and provide tranquillity.

Reflexes

Hands

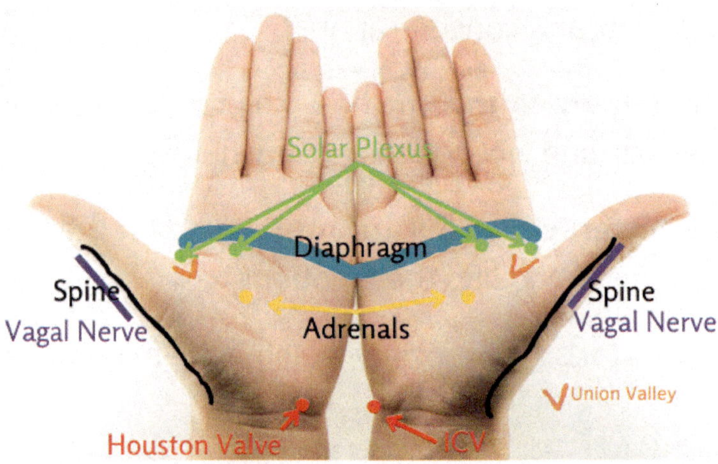

Along with the reflexes in the diagram you could include the digestion reflexes too.

Ear

Rub these points. If any feel sharp, keep rubbing. (See Chapter 9 for more information on working reflex points)

General points - ***Adrenals, Shen Men point*** - for anxiety, stress, and insomnia

Vagus nerve and Digestive points (as shown in the digestive image in the previous chapter)

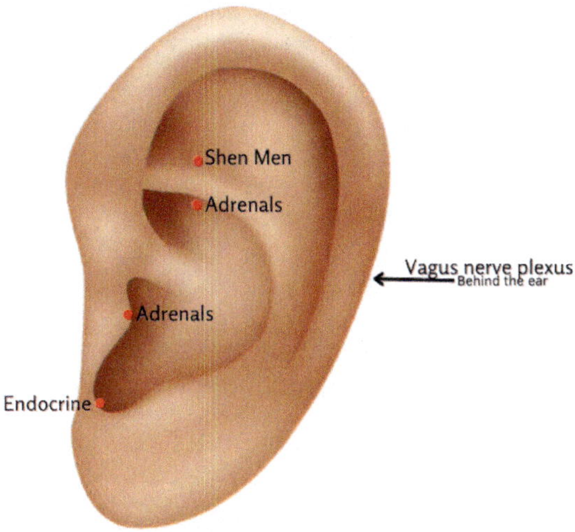

Anxiety - Master Cerebral, Tranquiliser Point, Occiput, Heart, Nervousness

Depression - Antidepressant points, Excitement point, Endocrine point, Occiput, Pineal Gland

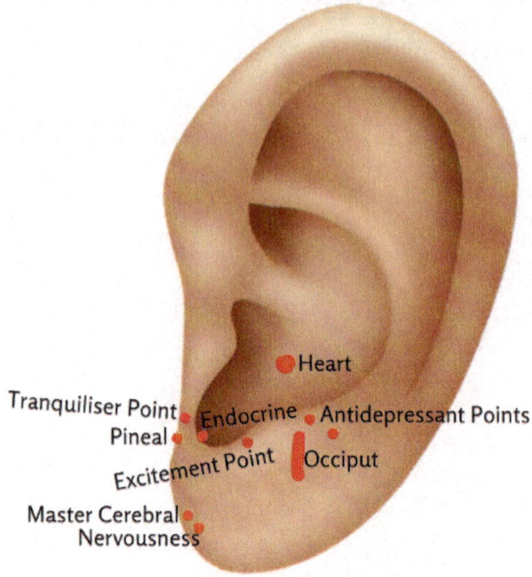

Memory and Concentration – Frontal cortex, Hippocampus, Memory, Master Cerebral, Heart

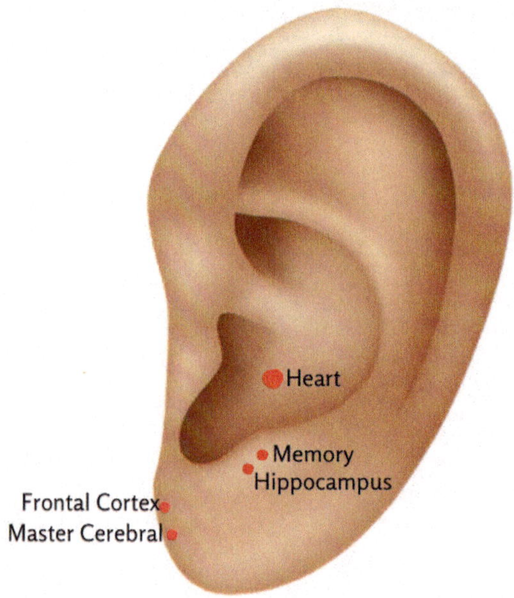

Face Yoga Routine

The Glabellar point – between brows and slightly above. Helps to balance the pineal gland that controls your body clock. So this point is also useful for sleep issues.

ESR or emotional stress response points are found mid forehead and in line with the pupils of eyes when looking forward. You probably hold your forehead naturally when you are anxious or you are trying to think and concentrate. Hold these points to defuse stress

Point Zero is found just in front of the ears. It is a reflexology point that is relaxing when you stroke down and stimulating when stroked up. For stress, anxiety, or before bed, rub up and down first. Then if you are feeling tired and fatigued during the day end with a few strokes going upwards. If you are wired and need to calm down finish with a few strokes going downwards.

Free the Hyoid. This small U-shaped bone is suspended in your throat and helps with chewing, swallowing, voice production, and tongue control. Unlike other bones, the hyoid is suspended and kept in place by ligaments and muscles. If you are stressed or anxious these muscles and ligaments become tight and the hyoid is unable to move freely to do its job. This often feels like you have something stuck in you throat and are unable to swallow. To free it up place your thumbs under your chin and firmly roll them round the rim of your jaw. You can also rub the other ends of the throat muscles down by the collarbone.

Chakras are also know as plexuses and are where two or more nerve cross and come together like an electrical junction box. These are very powerful to treat as they affect the organs each nerve runs to, nearby hormone glands, and their associated emotions. Chakras are found all over the body with the main 7 down the centre. On the face, these are represented down the middle of the face from the hairline to the tip of the nose, as seen in the diagram below. As you work these, be gentle. You can hold them, tap on them (to wake them up), or circle on them by planting your finger on to the skin and working both ways, moving the tissue not over the skin.

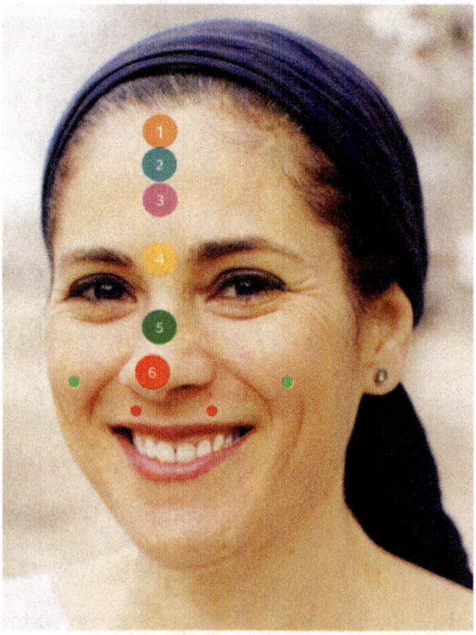

The other points in the diagram are the reflexology points for the adrenals and solar plexus. These are explained further in the next chapter on sleep.

For visual instructions, go to YouTube and explore the videos on my channel @serenitymojo7134

Rubbing Points

Around the navel is linked to the adrenals

Above and below the collarbone

Under the arms in the armpit

Inguinal lymph nodes in the crease of the upper thigh.

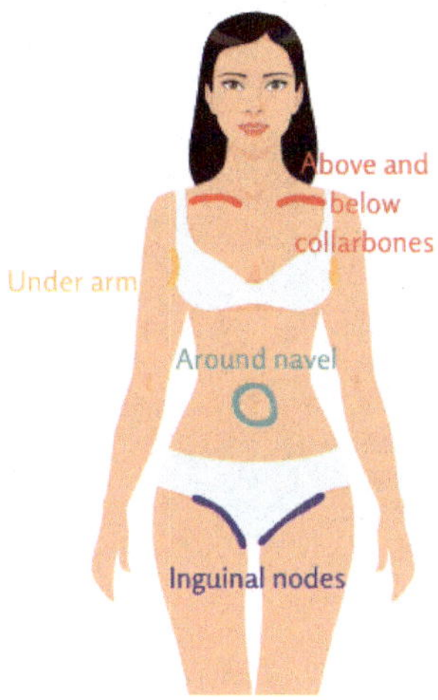

Movement

Exercise can stress the body and help it to relax. If you feel anxious and shaky during the day your cortisol levels may have increase. Try to use this up by running on the spot, taking a brisk walk, or doing some star jumps. This will lower your stress hormones and take you mind off what was stressing you out.

During perimenopause it is worth cutting down on your very high intensity exercise especially if you are not used to doing that kind of exercise. Listen to your body, if you feel exhausted during a gym session or a running, stop or slow down. We are all different. If your HPA axis is particularly sensitive now some intensive exercise may worsen your symptoms. Low-moderate intensity routines can lower cortisol while increasing your happy hormones, reducing pain, and lifting mood.

Daily activity to include into your day:

- A brisk walk or bike ride
- Cleaning the house
- Gardening
- Yoga
- Pilates
- Lion's Pose from the previous digestion chapter

Breathing

For anxiety and stress to calm emotions

Sit comfortably (or stand) in a quiet place

Inhale through your nose for a count of 4

Hold your breath for a count of 4

Exhale through your nose for a count of 4

Repeat for 2-3 minutes at the start increasing to 10 minutes after a few weeks.

Cooling breath to calm heat is excessive, leading to skin irritation, acidity, headaches, chronic pain, upset, or angry.

Sit comfortably

Extend your tongue past your lips and roll the sides upwards towards each other forming a tube shape. (Or open the mouth wide and stick out your tongue, curling the tip upwards)

Inhale through the curled tongue into the mouth like drinking through a straw.

Hold your breath for a comfortable length of time and exhale through both nostrils keeping the tongue extended. The exhale should be long, letting all the air out before inhaling again.

Repeat 3-5 times and then relax for 1 round.

You can repeat 5 rounds and then rest before completing another 5 rounds.

Heart coherence breathing

Find a comfortable and quiet place to sit or lie down

Place your hands over your heart area and breathe slow and deep

As you breathe, imagine that you are inhaling and exhaling through your heart

Focus on a positive emotion or memory that makes you feel calm, grateful, or happy

Try to maintain this state of heart coherence for at least five minutes

The benefits of heart coherence exercise include:

Reduced stress and anxiety

Enhanced immune system and cardiovascular health

Improved cognitive performance and creativity

Increased emotional balance and resilience

7

Tackle Your Sleep

As a baby you were trained to sleep through the night. Now it's time to bring back the adult bedtime routine!

Sleep quality is important at any age. It affects your mood, ability to concentrate and how you make sense of the world. While you sleep, your body is busy repairing tissues and taking out waste. During sleep your brain will receives a wash, clearing out harmful proteins. This is the only time your brain gets this vital wash! With you at rest, your body can take stock, adjust, and improve all its functions. Lack of sleep has been linked to a significantly higher risk of many medical conditions including obesity, type 2 diabetes, high blood pressure, heart disease and stroke.

Getting the best sleep quality is down to, you've guessed it, a balance of hormones. Changes in sleep patterns places your body under stress leading to low serotonin levels. This affects your mood, dreaming, vision and sleep patterns as well as influencing blood pressure, digestion, body temperature and pain.

If You do Nothing Else Get a Better Night's Sleep!

When you are tired, sleep deprived, and lacking energy the hormone Ghrelin is produced to tell your brain you are hungry and in need of energy, quickly. You are then programmed to seek out sugary and stodgy foods that are easy to break down. Once satisfied your body produces another hormone called Leptin to change the message to switch off the need for food. These natural hormone indicators can push you to overeat when your body constantly needs refuelling due to stress, lack of sleep, menopause chaos, or poor digestion. Are you getting the message and realising why this and the pervious chapters are in this book?

Your sleep-wake cycle is called your circadian rhythm or body clock. Each cell and the organ or structure they make up will have its own body clock. If one is running too slow the others are affected.

Sleep quality starts in the morning, getting light into the back of your eyes. Sitting by the window, going for a walk, or getting outside in the morning will reset your main clock controlled by the pineal gland. In the morning, light increases your cortisol levels to wake you up and get you moving. It also releases energy as it assumes you are going to be physically active. Mid-afternoon your cortisol levels decrease, and its hormone partner melatonin starts to increase. Melatonin starts to get you ready for sleep. Light starting to dim is another indicator that sleep time is coming.

An increase in light from screens and technology, vigorous and loud sounds, and fast activity will prolong high cortisol levels and stop the increase of melatonin. The result is not being able to get to sleep and/or waking up in the night.

During Perimenopause

During this time, it is even more important to manage your sleep. As progesterone declines and the balance between it and oestrogen and testosterone changes sleep is affected. Progesterone provides calmness affecting your sleep and mood.

You may be experiencing hot flushes (see symptom section for other tips). If this is the case, reduce your meat intake in the latter part of the day. Protein especially animal protein is heat inducing. Eat this in the morning and lunchtime. Keep you and your bedroom cool (see below).

Due to the fluctuating levels of oestrogen your digestion, heart rate and emotions may change too, causing disruption to your slumber. This is a common reason for holding or increasing weight. You may also have an increased risk of developing diabetes. Quit having added sugar, sugary drinks, alcohol, sugar in tea or coffee, fruit, and processed foods before bedtime and stop eating altogether after 8 pm. After this time insulin and blood sugar control is more difficult for your body leading it to producing more insulin. When insulin is high it depletes melatonin.

Other causes of sleep disruption in menopause include changes to your breathing, restless leg syndrome, some medication, emotional issues, or long-term illnesses.

Many perimenopausal women find that alcohol has differing effects on their body that lead to an intolerance. When it comes to sleep, alcohol makes you fall straight into a deep sleep state, skipping the REM sleep. Normally your will get 5-6 cycles of REM through the night where you will dream vividly, and power up your memory and concentration for the following day. By skipping some of these vital cycles you will be left with a groggy feeling the next morning, be more emotional throughout the day, and experience challenged brain function.

Tools for Better Sleep

- Develop a bed-time routine starting in the morning by getting light into the back of your eyes. You could go for a walk or eat your breakfast by a window.
- Be active during the morning and early afternoon. Your body is primed for this with higher cortisol levels.
- Eat your best meals early in the day. Your body can control blood sugars and insulin levels better in the morning than late at night. It can also digest the food better as it has more energy.
- In the evening start to wind down and slow your

movements. Incorporate a bed-time routine that involves as many of your senses as possible:

1. Reduce the light – This may include wearing blue light reducing glasses. Avoid flashing bright lights.

2. Calm the sounds – listen to slower more tranquil music.

3. Use the same essential oils to train your mind that sleep time is coming.

4. Make your bedroom a haven for sleep. Use the colours, the feel of your bedding and surroundings to teach your mind this is where you sleep and recharge.

5. Make sure your bed is comfortable. Changing your pillows and mattress can make a huge difference. Think about what type of bed and bedding you need, some are more cooling than others! Pillows wear out and can cause muscular problems that wake you up.

6. Keep your timings the same every day, even at the weekends. Decide what time you go to bed and what time you wake and get up.

Keep cool – your body temperature is vital for good quality sleep. If you are experiencing night sweats aim on cooling your head. Heat regulation occurs in a conversation between the thyroid, pituitary, and hypothalamus. During the peri-menopausal chaos and the lowering of oestrogen, the hypothalamus struggles to operate your thermostat. It triggers the cooling process by dilating blood vessels to remove heat from the surface of the skin. Your body is naturally warmer when blood pressure is higher (about 6-7.30 in the morning), and this is when most women say they have their hot flushes. It is important to get active straight away to burn off the cortisol and excess energy. One of the ways you can cool down a high temperature is to apply a cool cloth to your forehead or neck. You may want to blow cool air at your head or feet. I always stick my feet out of the duvet to keep my body temperature under control. Experiment yourself to find what works for you. There will be more hot flush reducing tools in the symptoms section.

Increase you melatonin – check you are getting enough carbs before bed, and also vitamin D, B6, B12, Zinc, Selenium, Magnesium, and Iron. You can check these levels with your medical professional or health practitioner. Some vitamins and minerals should not be taken as a supplement unless you really need them as they can cause an imbalance with another nutrient if you take too much. Other good sources of melatonin include fresh cranberries, bananas, walnuts, grains, mushrooms, or pistachio nuts 2-3 hours before bed.

Having a bath as part of your routine can be a great way to relax. You could jazz it up with some Epsom salts, which is a great way to increase your magnesium levels too. You could also add some diluted essential oils. Or if bathing is not your thing you could cool your body down with a cooling foot bath and add the Epsom salts and oils into that. This will help increase your magnesium, lower your body temperature, increase your brown fat activity helping weight loss, and improve your mental health! Love tools that have more than one effect!

Work on your breathing – snoring is actually more common in menopause. Obstructive sleep apnoea (OSA) is a sleeping disorder characterized by temporary pauses in breathing. This leads to gasping, snoring, choking sounds, and poor sleep quality usually due the lower progesterone levels. Practicing your breathing is more important, now. You can also use strips of tape to go over the mouth to ensure you are breathing through your nose and not your mouth. This small change can have huge benefits not only to your sleep but your overall health too.

Essential Oils

See Chapter 9 to check for cautions with individual oils, especially if you have medical conditions.

Chamomile, Roman - an insomnia oil that calms, soothes, and sedates. Is also said to help reduce temperature that causes sweating.

Frankincense – a lung oil that is warming and induces slow deep breathing. It will calm and comfort.

Jasmine – a relaxing, warm, and welcoming oil. Particularly useful in stressful times when on the edge of burnout.

Lavender – a calming, cheering, and balancing oil that helps when stressed. It is particularly good for nerve conditions either physically creating pain and discomfort or emotionally soothing sensitivities.

Mandarin – a light oil that helps revive and restore mental energy. Useful for emotional stress, anxiety, and insomnia.

Marjoram – a nurturing, soothing oil that is deeply relaxing and helpful for reducing emotional and physical responses.

Melissa (Lemon balm) – an anxiety reducing oil that is good for insomnia and nerve pains. Particularly good when over-anxious and concerned about other.

Patchouli – a grounding oil that help the mind to be more objective. If you are feeling weepy, moody, indecisive, and oversensitive this is for you.

Rose – a beautiful female oil that is gentle and balancing. Use when love and kindness to yourself and others is needed.

Sandalwood – another deep breathing oil that is comforting, soothing and creates a sense of peace. It is meditative, serene and a great oil for insomnia.

Valarian – not the best smelling oil (like sweaty socks!) but a knockout oil. Just remember to blend it well to hide the smell.

Vetiver – sedating, grounding, tranquil and extremely relaxing, like a pre-med before an operation.

Ylang Ylang – a sensual, balancing oil that calms the heart and slows the breath.

Reflexes

Feet

Use a ball or cooled water bottle underneath the foot and rub along the spine and underside of the foot.

Ear

Rub these points. If any feel sharp, keep rubbing. (See Chapter 9 for more information on working reflex points)

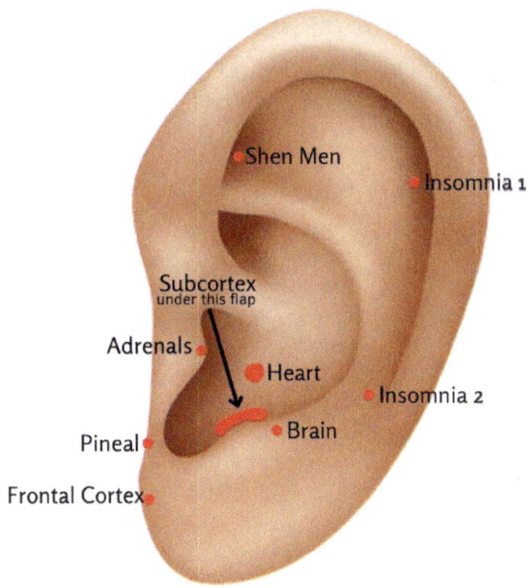

Face Yoga Routine

Prepare for bed using jaw rubbing, particularly if you are a teeth grinder. This will benefit your jaw and the rest of your body as it calms the nervous system especially the vagal nerve and works to loosen the connective tissue.

Solar plexus – find the lowest part of the cheekbones with your thumbs and push up

Adrenals – find the roots of your incisors with fingertips and hold or rotate on this point

Chakras/plexuses – a plexus is a junction box of nerves and there are 7 main ones down the centre of the body. 6 of these can be picked up on the face. Each have associated glands and are shown on the diagram below. Starting with plexus number 1 plant and rotate a finger on the point clockwise and then anticlockwise. Use small circles without sliding on the skin but moving the tissue.

1. Pineal, pituitary, and hypothalamus

2. Thyroid and parathyroid

3. Thymus

4. Pancreas

5. Adrenals

6. Ovaries

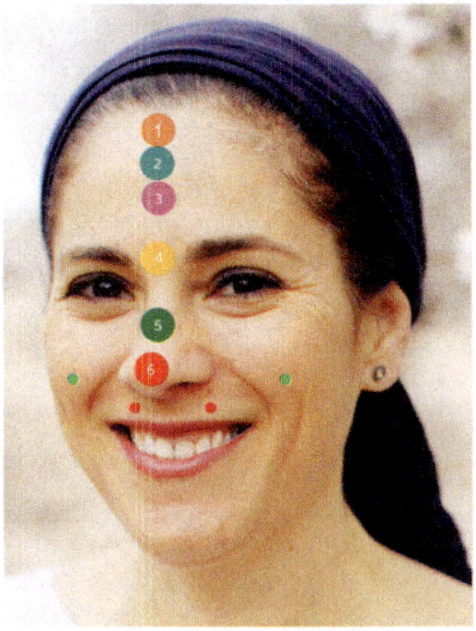

For visual instructions, go to YouTube and explore the videos on my channel @serenitymojo7134

Rubbing Points

Tensor Fascia Lata (TFL), around the pubic bone (very gently), 5cm (2") above and sides of the navel, and the Angle of Louis (the flat bone at the top of the breastbone.

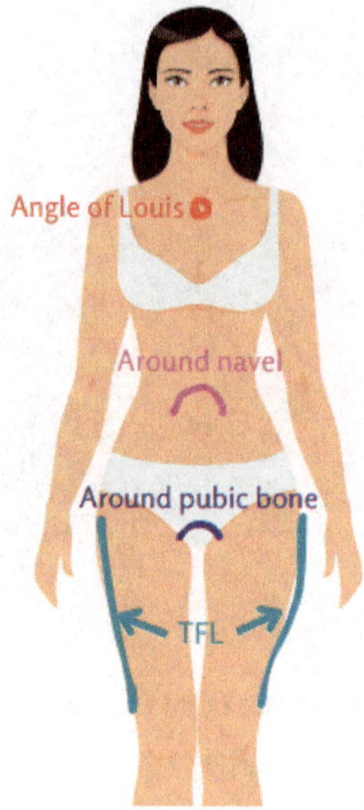

If breathing is an issue or you consistently wake between 3-5 am, rub between ribs 3-5 and go back to sleep

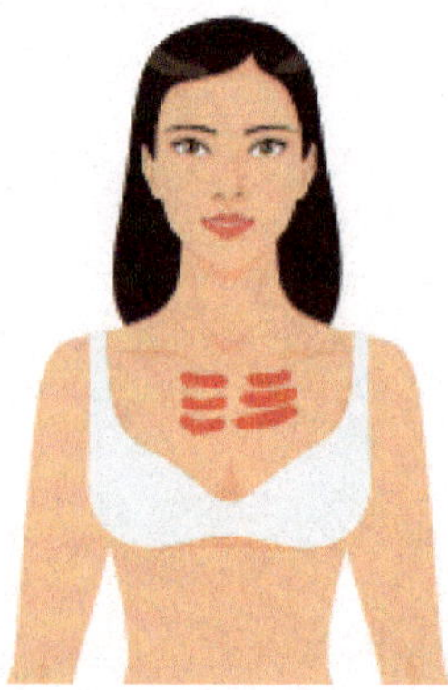

If you wake consistently between 1-3am or have been drinking alcohol rub GB31 and between the 5-6 ribs on the right. GB31 is found by standing with your hands hanging down

the sides of your legs. The point is where the tip of your middle finger touches is GB31.

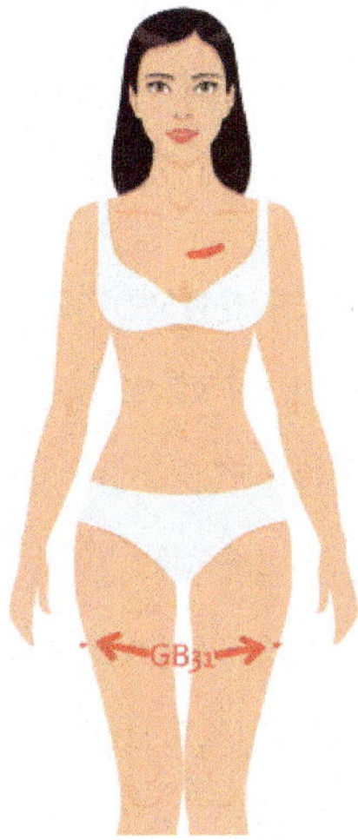

If you are awake between 5-7am rub Tensor Fascia Lata (TFL), Inner thigh, and hipbone crest (ASIC).

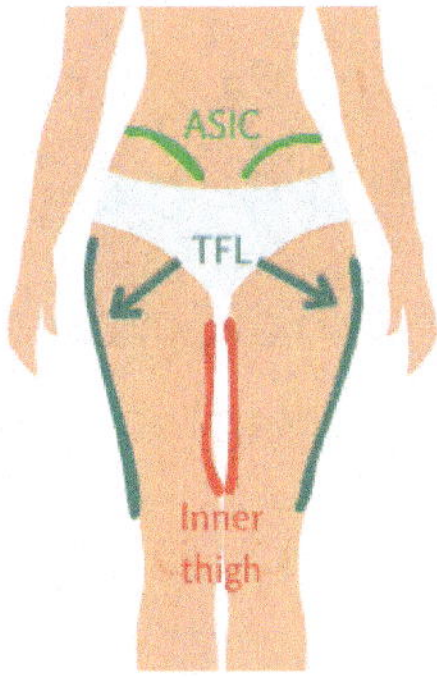

Movement

A stretch before bed is the best time for your body. When you are asleep your body is stationery and stiffness can become more obvious. Deep slow stretching and movement before bed will help relax and remove muscle tension. Light stretching and joint movement when you wake will help flush out any stiffness formed during the night.

Breathing

As I have said before, it is important to practice breathing through your nose particularly in your sleep. It turns out that mouth breathing affects 'the levels of carbon dioxide and oxygen in the bloodstream' according to Dr Burhenne. He and other dentists talk about mouth taping where you place a small piece of cloth tape over closed relaxed lips before sleep. This trains you to become a nose breather while you sleep. Make sure the tape you use is gentle enough to remove in the morning.

Set your phone or alarm to prompt you to check you are breathing through your nose during the day as this has huge health benefits too (references – Breath by James Nestor, Ask the dentist, and sleep foundation)

Best breathing techniques to do before bed are those that relax you. With modern technology you can do these with or without relaxation music.

My rib cage breathing (you could also use belly or abdominal breathing)

Sit or lie comfortably and without changing anything, notice your breath.

As you breath in through your nose notice the front of your ribcage lift and expand. Then fall as you breath out. Repeat for a couple more breaths.

Now, as you breath in expand the rib cage out to the sides and notice it fall as you breath out. Repeat for a couple more breaths.

Next as you breath in push the back of your ribs out and then watch the back ribs fall as you breath out. Repeat for a couple more breaths.

Now put it all together and fully expand the ribcage out as you breath is and relax as you breath out. Repeat for 20 breaths before relaxing and breathing normally again.

Breathing with the whole ribcage moves the diaphragm and along with it all the organs of you abdomen like your kidneys, liver, stomach, intestines. It releases the fascia holding it all up and pumps the lymph clearing the waste more efficiently.

Another technique:

I often find some people tense up and breath quicker as soon as you focus on your breath. So, you may like to listen to some relaxation music or guided imagery. My only stipulation is you breathe through your nose!

8

Alleviating Your Symptoms

Emotional Symptoms

Brain fog, poor concentration, anxiety and panicky, memory lapse, irritability, mood swings, dizziness.

What is Happening?

Oestrogen and testosterone levels are fluctuating, while progesterone levels are slowly declining. Oestrogen affects brain clarity, memory, and concentration. Testosterone affects the speed and sharpness of the brain. Progesterone has a calming effect and lack of this hormone is probably the most common reason for increased anxiety. As progesterone decreases, cortisol can rise making you feel more stressed and agitated. Feeling more anxious and panicky will also have an effect sleep, memory, mood, and concentration.

The changes happening, affect the blood vessels to the brain, bringing fresh nutrients and clearing out waste. Fluctuating oestrogen affects the production of serotonin in the brain and intestines, which affects dopamine levels.

Where to Start?

Taking control of your stress levels is most important for your health and wellbeing through perimenopause and beyond. Make sure your sleep quality in at its best too. Through perimenopause you can expect emotions and brain function to vary with your fluctuating hormones. Reducing your stress is key to making these symptoms as mild as possible. This means eating nourishing foods in a mindful way, lowering the intensity of your exercise when tired, and overall listening to your body. If you feel weary, take time out to rest and relax or better still build this into your daily life.

DIM from cruciferous vegetables help the body to detoxify excess oestrogen while flaxseed and their oil are a natural progesterone. Remember that hormones respond to each other and are never static. They change from day to day, hour to hour, minute by minute.

Using the right essential oils, breathing techniques, and doing small things you enjoy daily are a good place to start with your emotions. Get the basics right like having a wash, getting dressed, putting on your face creams and a bit of make up, brushing your hair, even making your bed. These will all make you feel a little better and in time improve your mood and energy.

Insomnia and Fatigue

What is Happening?

Sleep issues occur due to the disruption of other symptoms like sweats, increased heartbeat, palpitations, aches and pains or urinary issues. These need to be addressed individually.

Changes in producing melatonin, your sleepy hormone, and changes in the effectiveness of your digestion can lead to deficiencies in nutrients like magnesium and the calming B vitamins.

When you sleep well, growth hormone is restored. This controls your appetite hormones. Leptin which tells your brain you are full and keeps insulin low while you sleep. If you wake up in the night or early in the morning, feeling hungry this could be the cause.

Where to Start?

Improving the efficiency of your digestion and absorption will supply your body with the ingredients for combating stress, sleep issues, and emotional health. Feeding your gut bacteria will reward you with vital nutrients and happy hormones. Eat food containing plenty of B vitamins like wholegrains, legumes, green leafy vegetables, nuts, and seeds. Remember marvellous magnesium and use Epsom salts in your bath. Read through the sleep chapter for more information and tips.

Headaches (or migraines)

What is Happening?

Headaches can be structural, emotional, biochemical (from food or chemical sensitivities) or hormonal. You may need to think about seeking the advice from your doctor, or treatments with kinesiologist, nutritionist, or physical therapist like a masseur, sports therapist, osteopath, or chiropractor.

Changes in hormones, especially when oestrogen declines can trigger a headache or migraine. Many women who suffer monthly migraines report that they decline through and beyond menopause! Everyone is different.

You may be over tired with anxiety or sleep issues, dehydrated after hot flushes and night sweats, or be unable to flush out toxins as your liver is working extremely hard at this time with its increased workload. Check out and work on these areas. You may need to rule out any thyroid issues. This gland helps out the other glands especially when they are tired.

Where to Start?

Look after your liver and help your lymphatic system to reduce your toxic load. Keep reading to find out how to reduce your hot flushes and make sure you are drinking enough water. Your hydration levels also includes consuming fewer dehydrating foods and drinks like tea, coffee, alcohol, salty and dried foods. You can also increase foods full of water like lettuce, cucumber, cruciferous vegetables, melon, citrus fruits, and berries.

Remember rubbing and releasing your jaw is a great for releasing tension. Daily treatment will help your sleep, deal with the stress cycle and so much more.

Take care of yourself with relaxing treatments and seek advice from a professional.

Hot flushes and Night sweats

You may have noticed changes in sweat and body odour. These symptoms are very common. Some women do not experience flushes and sweats while others continue with them post menopause when periods have finished. With that in mind this section is a little longer.

What is Happening?

The cause of hot flushes and night sweats are not entirely understood, however this is what we do know:

- The hypothalamus is the body's thermostat. When oestrogen is in short supply the parameters of your core body temperature becomes narrower. This means that the hypothalamus may interpret 37 degrees C as overheating and instruct the body to sweat as a way of cooling down.

- These symptoms are also linked to anxiety, thoughts and panic feelings which set off a sweating response.
- Body odour can change due to the changes in yeast on the surface of the skin and your immune system.

Where to Start?

It is thought that a hot flush starting at the toes and zip up very fast are the result of lowering progesterone levels creating too much cortisol. If this is you, look at controlling your blood sugars and your stress first.

If your hot flushes start in the middle of your body and radiate out in a sweat lasting up to 10 minutes, your oestrogen levels may be too low. You may also have vaginal dryness and be very forgetful.

Reducing stress and having some time to relax every day is so important. This includes diaphragmatic or another type of breathing exercise.

Identify what triggers your flush, for example:

- Stress or anxious thoughts
- Spicy foods
- Coffee or alcohol
- Wearing clothing that's too warm for the environment

- Having a high temperature
- Smoking
- Medical treatments and drugs
- Other health conditions, like diabetes, tuberculosis, or an overactive thyroid
- Types of cancer treatment

Make the necessary adjustments to your eating and drinking, clothing, or if medical, consult your doctor and see if they can suggest changes.

Here are some lifestyle suggestions to try:

- Avoid your known triggers, such as spicy foods, MSG foods, alcohol, and caffeine. It could be something else but these are the most common.
- If possible quit smoking, or avoid second hand smoke
- Avoid added simple sugars and eating after 8pm
- Dress in layers so that it is easy to remove a layer if a hot flush occurs
- Carry water with ice, if possible, to sip at when a hot flush begins
- Use a portable fan and take it with you
- Keep your bedroom cool at night

- Avoid high intensive exercise immediately before bedtime
- Practice deep breathing and relaxation exercises daily
- Establish your own calming routine to reduce stress, especially before bed
- Follow a healthy eating plan, getting regular exercise to reach or maintain a healthy weight
- Post-menopause eat a serving of soy each day to decrease hot flashes and their intensity. The soy must be good quality and not over processed. Soy can interact with some medications, so check it is safe for you before taking.
- Black cohosh supplements or oil used short term have been used for the treatment of hot flushes and night sweats (these can cause digestive irritation, abnormal bleeding, or blood clots and should not be used if your liver is struggling)
- Evening primrose supplements or oil can treat hot flushes (EPO can cause nausea or diarrhoea and if you are on medication check with your doctor before taking)
- Add ground flaxseeds to your salads, breakfast etc or take flax supplements or oil (also known as linseed)

- Eat foods containing Vitamin B and E

Tissue changes

Including stress incontinence, more urinary infections, vaginal dryness, muscle or joint pain and stiffness, prickly skin, itchy skin, dry and thinning skin and hair, dry eyes, brittle nails, facial hair, restless leg syndrome, dry or burning mouth, gum disease or ulcers, tinnitus, breast soreness

What is Happening?

All tissues, like muscles, skin, hair, and nails are affected by the changes in oestrogen levels.

Oestrogen plays a big part in the production of collagen and elastin that keeps your tissues supple and elastic. Without oestrogen, all internal tissues including blood and lymph vessels, digestive muscles, heart, etc become more rigid and less flexible. When flexibility is compromised, the texture of the tissue changes. This can lead to inflammation in an area and more chance of infection.

During perimenopause the immune system can be lowered and/or nutrient deficiencies occur creating these problems too. Sometimes the body uses up certain nutrients creating a nutrient deficiency, or it may occur if your digestion is not working efficiently enough. The deficiency will depend on your general health, stress levels, where you are in your menopause journey, your lifestyle, and your sleep quality.

A change in the steroid hormone levels will cause the vaginal and urinary tissue to become thinner and more irritated. Sex and urination may become painful with a greater chance of thrush.

Where to Start?

Addressing your digestion is key, to make sure you are eating well, digesting well, and absorbing well.

Getting movement in the vaginal and urinary area is a must. Pelvic floor exercises are important to do at any age but especially now. Hopefully you use a moisturiser on your face and neck or may a body cream. Now is the time to add the use of a vaginal moisturiser. Yes, they do exist! Make sure you find one that is good quality, gentle and without irritants or fragrances.

It is important to stretch well after exercise. Keep changing the way you move and stretch to work all the muscles, joints, ligaments, and nerves. This will also keep your lymph system flowing efficiently to get rid of the waste and prevent build up in joints, muscles, and skin. The lymph system is so important for the smooth running and health of the whole body especially your immune system, hormone balancing, and brain function.

Your skin, hair, and nails reflect your overall health. However, to help internally, eat plenty of foods containing antioxidants (vitamin A, C, D, E, CoQ10, and good oils). Working on the outside use good quality personal care products that have high levels of organic ingredients and massage them in well. Rub any virgin oil or hoof ointment used on animal's hooves to rub into your cuticles and over you nails. Just like your body, your face needs a combination of massage, exercise, and lymphatic drainage. There are face yoga tips throughout this book aimed at each chapter and if you look on my YouTube channel, @SerenityMojo, you will find some classes there too. You could use your favourite light face oil to enhance your face yoga sessions.

Mouth conditions are more common if your immune system is compromised. This is more likely with higher stress levels. Teeth and mouth tissue also need plenty of saliva. This is the first stage in the fight against invaders like bacteria. Saliva is mainly water (so drink plenty), and its production is stimulated by eating and chewing. When your mouth is dry avoid things like coffee, soda, alcohol, spicy and salty foods. Visiting the dentist to make sure your teeth are aligned can help not only mouth health but can stop you grinding your teeth and jaw clenching too.

That leads us neatly to your jaw and its importance. Chewing is discussed in the Chapter about your digestion and there are links to face yoga techniques to help release the jaw on my YouTube channel @SerenityMojo. The joints of the jaw, (the TMJ) can account for many of the symptoms put down as menopausal. These include tinnitus, vertigo, dizziness, oral diseases, fatigue, irritability, headaches, migraines, depression, anxiety, brain fog, insomnia, dry eyes, visual disturbances, light sensitivity, joint and muscle aches, and pains etc. Working to balance your TMJ in menopause is important. When changes occur to the oestrogen production the alveolar bone decreases causing gum inflammation and possible teeth loss. Tightening of the jaw joints can happen with the triggering of the stress response which will drive more stress in a continuous cycle. Go back to the chapter on stress to find out what your triggers are.

Joint and Bone health

This follows on from tissue changes as the same information applies here. Many women start to worry about bone health, finding their joints are becoming more stiff, sore, and even painful.

What is Happening?

Apart from the adjustment in oestrogen levels, your recovery time after exercise or an active day become slower in peri-menopause. If you add to this poor sleep (when healing and repair happens), and changes to joint lubrication your risk of injuries increase. As discussed previously, the lymph vessels that clear out waste and the blood vessels that bring energy and healing are prone to stiffness too. This compromises their function.

Where to Start?

Make sure you have read the chapters on sleep, stress, and lymph (and digestion) to understand how to optimise these areas. If your sleep is poor at the moment, lower the intensity of your exercise and incorporate gentle joint mobilising movements daily. Keep your cortisol levels in check by working on your sleep quality and stress levels.

Eat more beetroot and celery or put them in your juices and smoothies. These help to dilate blood vessels. Remember to check if you are on medication before starting.

Add antioxidants into your diet, these are important going forward too. Basically, make sure you are eating plenty of fruit and vegetables. These are not only full of antioxidants but gut bacteria feeding fibre too. If you are kind to your gut bacteria, they will provide you with Vitamin K which will ensures calcium reaches your bones and teeth. That's what I can a win win!

Eat mainly alkaline forming foods like green leafy vegetables and ensure you are having enough folate, B vitamins, and marvellous magnesium.

Make sure you are having plenty of good oils like olive oil. Oils are especially important to your health now and good omega 3 oils help to get rid of inflammation from bad fats. Remember, oils are not the enemy. They provide vital nutrients like A, D, E and K, that protect your tissues from degrading.

Collagen supplements are all the rage these days. There are different types of collagen throughout the body. Vitamin C and D are important for maintaining type 1 so sunlight and brightly colour foods are key. In supplement form, read the ingredients carefully. Best source for joints and bones is collagen hydrolysate.

Other nutrients that help your joints and bones include:

- Glucosamine and chondroitin
- MSM – a source of sulphur and great for cartilage, hair, skin, and nails
- Manganese, boron, and silicon are trace minerals, so if you are thinking about taking these as a supplement check with a nutrition specialist or if on medication your healthcare team.
- Vitamin D3 and K2 together build for strong bones

Digestive changes

Including bloating, constipation, weight gain, and sensitivities

By now you have plenty of knowledge about your digestion and how to combat these symptoms but just to recap.

What is Happening?

During the menopause hormone chaos many of the changes effect on your digestion. For a while you may become sensitive to foods you have not previously, the gut lining may change, and there may be more demand for certain nutrients that make it appear you are deficient.

Of course, all these symptoms can be experienced at any age but with the increase in the liver's workload they may become more acute.

As your body changes where it gets oestrogen from, and the type of oestrogen produced changes too. This makes you more prone to gaining weight around the middle. Progesterone levels declines at a constant rate over time while oestrogen levels fluctuate creating at times an imbalance between the two. When this happens, and particularly if the detox organs are overstretched (and your stress levels are high), the excess oestrogen is stored. The preferred areas to store it are your abdomen and breast area.

Where to Start?

Make sure you control your stress, relax your jaw, love your liver and lymph, eat more fibre, and reduce your sugar. Read all the previous chapters!

Heart Health

You may be more aware of irregular heartbeat or palpitations due to oestrogen levels. Although this does not mean a problem, it may be worth checking if you are concerned.

What is Happening?

Oestrogen protects the heart and blood vessels. As mentioned before, it also keeps blood vessels and heart muscles flexible. If you are overweight, have high blood pressure or a family history or you have an autoimmune disease, your heart disease risk factor may have increased.

Where to Start?

Exercise and movement is important. Eating plenty of fish, flaxseeds, fruit, nuts, and vegetables, and reducing sugary foods and drinks

Menstrual cycle

During perimenopause one of the first symptoms, you may notice are changes to your cycle. They may be heavier, more painful, more frequent, longer, or lighter and less frequent.

What is Happening?

Menstruation may be unpredictable while your body adjusts to the new hormone levels. In a cycle, before menopause, the release of progesterone after ovulation contracts the uterine blood vessels limiting bleeding. In perimenopause, when ovulation is irregular and progesterone is low, this can result in heavy bleeding.

If heavy bleeding is constant, check with your doctor.

Where to Start?

Be prepared! Make a pack of things you need for menstruation and carry it with you at all times. This may include sanitary products, pain killers, essential oil blends etc

Remember this phase is not for ever and it will pass.

Libido

Low libido is very common, and you may need to educate your partner to the chaos of menopause so that they understand.

What is Happening?

Caused by lower oestrogen and testosterone levels. After menopause these are produced by the adrenals. Remember, if stress levels are high these hormone levels will be low as your body will make more stress hormones.

A decrease in pleasure neurotransmitters like serotonin, dopamine and histamine will reduce motivation and arousal.

Where to Start?

Make sure you and your partner are a team on this. Find other pleasurable pursuits that keep the bond between you strong.

By now you will have picked up on the importance of controlling stress levels (it affects all your symptoms in some way). Find time for solitary relaxation as well as time together. Most of your serotonin comes from your gut so digestion is important as well as good sleep. If you find intercourse painful, see the solutions above for vaginal dryness and talk to your partner.

An organic vaginal moisturiser or lubricant can be used whether you are on HRT or not and will help you feel more comfortable.

Aphrodisiac essential oils include:

- Sweet basil
- Black pepper
- Cedarwood
- Chamomile Maroc
- Cinnamon coriander – euphoric
- Ginger
- Jasmine
- Juniper berry
- Marjoram sweet
- Neroli
- Patchouli
- Pine, scotch
- Rose otto
- Rosewood
- Sandalwood

- Savory summer
- Thyme – Moroccan, common red or white – mental sexual tonic
- Vetiver
- Ylang ylang

Have fun experimenting with those that work for your and blend them in one or a blend of these carrier oils – Sunflower, Borage, Jojoba, or Vitamin E

9

Holistic Remedies Explained

Holistic remedies work by balancing the body and reducing the stress load so that your body can do what it does best – keep you safe, functioning well, and returning you to health. Over time, your body may struggle to get the resources it needs or find the energy to complete this task. When this happens, eat well, hydrate, rest and keep using the techniques in this book.

Essential Oils and Cautions

Essential oils are natural extracts from plants that have various benefits for your health and wellness. For the plant, they are the immune system protecting it from predators and diseases. They also send messages and activate functions in the plant like hormones for us as well as provide an internal transport system like blood in mammals.

They can be used in different ways, such as aromatherapy treatments, massage, skincare, cleaning and more. However, true essential oils are very concentrated and potent, so need to be used with care and caution. You need to think of essential oils as highly concentrated substances where less is more.

All essential oils are:

- ***Oxygenating*** – they act as oxygen donors allowing cells to breathe and therefore help in the formation of new skin or tissue cells.
- ***Detoxifying*** – have cleansing and antibacterial qualities that clear and clean waste matter out of the body.
- ***Volatile*** – they evaporate in the open air, hence why inhalation is a good method of use. A suitable blend will be smell pleasant to you. Odours affect various parts of the brain. The **limbic** system is associated with emotional memories and may trigger a childhood memory, feelings, sexual arousal, food appetite and body temperature.

Always dilute essential oils before applying them to your skin or inhaling them. For this you can use a carrier oil, like coconut, almond, jojoba, or olive oil. A general rule of thumb is to use 1-2 drops of essential oil per teaspoon of carrier oil.

If you are on medication or have sensitive skin, check with your doctor or an aromatherapist for any complications. You could do a patch test before using a new essential oil. To do this apply a small amount of the diluted oil to a discreet area of your skin, like the inside of your elbow or wrist, and wait for 24 hours. If you experience any redness, itching, burning, or swelling, wash off immediately with water and discontinue use. If the reaction is extreme consult your doctor.

Avoid using essential oils on children, pregnant or breast-feeding women, pets, or people with medical conditions without consulting a doctor or a certified aromatherapist first. Some essential oils may have adverse effects on these groups of people or interfere with medications. See the guide below too.

Store your oils in a cool, dark, dry place away from direct sunlight, heat, and moisture. Keep them out of reach of children and pets. Do not ingest essential oils unless directed by a doctor or a certified aromatherapist.

Learn about the properties and effects of different essential oils before blending them. Some essential oils may complement each other well, while others may clash or cancel each other out. Also think about the time of day you are using them and what you will be doing after use. For example, avoid using a heavy sedating oil like vetiver if you are about to drive or first thing in the morning. Some oils have a cooling effect like peppermint, while others are warming like ginger. So if you are having hot flushes ginger will not be the best oil. You can use online resources or books to find out more about the characteristics and benefits of each essential oil and how to blend them harmoniously. You will find a list of my favourites at the back of the book.

Experiment with different combinations and ratios of essential oils to create your own unique blends. You can use a diffuser, an inhaler, a spray bottle, a roller bottle, or a tissue to enjoy your blends. Label your blends with the names and amounts of the essential oils you used for future reference.

If you would like to learn more about how to choose and blend your own oil products to use at home sign up for my course here

Check Your Cautions

Basil sweet – If high in Methyl Chavicol, avoid with high blood pressure. Avoid in pregnancy.

Benzoin – is very relaxing effect so do not use when concentration is necessary.

Bergamot – if it contains Bergapten, Bergamot is phototoxic, but you can buy it without this chemical. Regular use has the risk of being carcinogenic. Oxidised oils or those containing high levels of d-limonene increase the sensitising effects. Otherwise, this oil is treated as a citrus and is non-toxic.

Black pepper – Skin irritant and overuse can cause kidney damage.

Cedarwood – best to be avoided in pregnancy as it is very strong and may be a skin irritant.

Chamomile maroc – Moroccan chamomile contains 1,8 cineole, which gives it a sweet smell, and alpha pinene, which is a mild dermal irritant.

Chamomile, German and Roman – none known

Cinnamon leaf – Never apply to your face and use with care as it can irritate the skin and mucous membranes. Avoid in pregnancy.

Clary sage – Can induce drowsiness so avoid high dosage when you must drive. Avoid with anti-depressants and alcohol. SCLAREOL (an alcohol) has oestrogen type properties, so should be avoid in hormone related cancers.

Clove bud – a very potent oil so use with care (below 1drop in a teaspoon). Can cause mucus membrane irritation. Avoid in pregnancy.

Coriander – Can stupefy in large doses

Cypress – Nontoxic

Dill – avoid if taking medication and do not use oil that has been oxidised.

Eucalyptus – Avoid with high BP, epilepsy & homeopathic formulas.

Eucalyptus, blue gum – None known

Fennel, sweet – Not to be used with epileptic, in pregnancy, or with children. Generally, for mature people and should be used in moderation.

Frankincense – Due to the content of some unknown chemicals avoid during pregnancy.

Geranium – Avoid in early pregnancy. High in alcohols and esters making it open to adulteration. Can cause allergic reaction to those specifically allergic to geraniums.

Ginger – Not to be used in acid and heartburn conditions.

Grapefruit – This oil does not appear to be phototoxic. Do not use with time release heart medication.

Hyssop – Avoid in pregnancy and epilepsy

Jasmine – is deeply relaxing and should be used in small quantities or it may impair concentration. Avoid in pregnancy.

Juniper – A strong diuretic – do not use in the first few months of pregnancy; things may get worse before they get better (healing crisis risk) Will lower the blood sugar levels – be careful with diabetics, make them aware to check their blood over next 24 hours.

Juniper Sabina is a skin irritant & abortive.

Juniper, Common and alpine should be avoided when using on damaged or sensitive skin. Causes urine & water retention if used in large amounts or too regularly – avoid using with kidney disease, acute kidney, and bladder infection.

Lavender, true – overuse can over stimulate the nervous system, take care with epilepsy

Lemon – phototoxic, avoid the sun when on the skin.

Lemongrass - can irritate sensitive skin and should be avoided in pregnancy

Lime - phototoxic, avoid the sun when on the skin.

Mandarin and Bitter orange - Can cause photosensitivity. Do not go outside when applied for at least 48 hours.

Marjoram, sweet - May lower blood pressure so do not use if yours is already low. Long-term use can deaden emotions and very sedative, meaning changing the oil is important. Avoid in pregnancy and use with care.

Melissa (lemon balm) - may cause skin irritation so to do not use more than 2 drops in a teaspoon. Avoid in pregnancy.

Myrrh - this soothing can become toxic in high doses and should be avoided in pregnancy.

Neroli - This oil is very calming so use with care when concentration is needed.

Niaouli - none known

Orange, bitter - phototoxic, avoid the sun when on the skin.

Orange, sweet - may be phototoxic, avoid the sun when on the skin.

Oregano - is a dermal toxin, skin irritant and mucus membrane irritant so it is best defused or blending 1 drop in 2 teaspoons of carrier. Avoid in pregnancy, breast-feeding and children under 7.

Palma Rosa - none known

Patchouli – Some people find this oil very overpowering, and some may find a loss of appetite, some care is needed when you use this oil.

Peppermint and spearmint – overuse can cause sleep pattern disturbances avoid with heart problems and homeopathic remedies. May irritant mucous membrane or irritate skin in high quantities. Away dilute, use in small quantities, (under 3 drops per teaspoon and no more) and do not ingest.

Petitgrain – can be a skin irritant under the influence of sunlight and may cause allergic reactions.

Ravensara – Ravensara is a good antiviral and viral preventer but can be a skin irritant.

Rose otto – none known

Rosemary – Verbenone and camphor chemotype should be avoided in pregnancy & not used on children due to verbenone (a ketone). Nb no formal testing has been carried out. Camphor type oils should be avoided with epilepsy. All types should be avoided with high blood pressure. If ingested a teaspoon may cause illness in an adult, an ounce may cause death.

Sage – this has high Ketone content which is Neurotoxic. Is abortive (although this is not proven) and not to be used in pregnancy and babies (0-5 months).

Sandalwood – may cause a skin rash on hypersensitive skins

Tea tree – Trees grown in northern Australia have a higher terpinene - 4 - ol than trees grown in the south and a lower cineole content. Cineole is a strong cold relief but is a mucus membrane and skin irritant (not good for healing wounds and inflammation). Terpinene - 4 - oil is the active principal in the treatment of AIDS.

Thyme common, sweet – avoid with high blood pressure or during pregnancy until the onset of labour.

Valarian – only use in very small doses as can have a very strong effect.

Ylang ylang - can cause nausea and headaches if used for too long.

Reflexes

Reflexology, as a treatment is deeply relaxing and wonderful for this stage of life. There are now many techniques that focus on balancing hormones, improving the lymphatic drainage, digestion, and urinary systems. There are many theories about how reflexology works and a growing number of scientific papers showing what effect it has on the body. Some of that research has been on foot reflexology and sleep disorders in menopausal women, vasomotor complaints (hot flushes), and depression. You can find links in the interesting reading section of the book.

Self-treating on your feet can be tricky, but working on the hands, face, and/or ears can be a start and enhance your treatments with a therapist. As hormones constantly fluctuate, daily self-treating helps to smooth out this transition. In each chapter of this book, you have been given specific reflexes to work. If you are not used to working with your hands in this way, there are tools to help you. The main aim is to stimulate the reflexes but not hurt yourself. Reaction to your treatment can vary from person to person. Some of the reflexes may feel tender. After working many reflexes, you may feel tired, have a release of emotions, or find that you have increased urination. Any physical or emotional changes, up to 24 hours after your self-care treatment is helped by drinking plenty of water and getting some rest. Symptoms sometimes get worse before they get better, therefore wait until you are feeling better and carry on.

The ears are used by reflexologist, chiropractors, and acupuncturists. All the systems of the body are mapped out on to the ears. As the ears are attached to the side of the head they are particularly linked to the cranial nerves, and the blood and lymph vessels between the head, jaw, and the rest of the body. The cranial nerves, send and receive messages with information from the skin, digestion, sight, sound, smell etc. This may include pain and discomfort, dangers, and internal or external stressors. Remember these nerve messages are received and analysed by the hypothalamus and action is taken when hormone messages are sent out to the relevant gland. Working the ears is easy and effective. The points of the ears only react when something needs to be addressed. Don't be surprised if your ear go red and hot – this is a great reaction as tension is being released. Work both ears for 5-10 minutes. Give an extra rub to any area that is tender or sharp to touch.

Face Yoga

Face yoga is a technique that involves exercises, acupressure, and massage techniques for your face, neck, and scalp. The idea is to tone the weakened facial muscles, relax the tense muscles and nerves, and improve the lymph drainage of the face and neck. The result is a smoothing of fine lines, better blood circulation, and healthier skin. Face yoga does not require any products, but it does require regular practice and isometric resistance.

Facial reflexology is particularly easy to incorporate into your daily face yoga routine. You can add some reflexology, face yoga, and lymph drainage massage techniques while you apply your moisturiser, oil, or serum in the morning or at night. You will gain all the benefits of stimulating the reflexes and be treating your skin, toning muscles, reducing puffiness, and helping you feel better about yourself too. Or you could use these techniques dry and over your make up while taking a break in the middle of the day.

Some of the benefits of face yoga and reflexology include:

- Release of tension, which can minimize the appearance of stress lines
- Strengthen and tone facial muscles to ultimately widen eyes, raise cheeks, and firm up the jawline

- Increase circulation and blood flow to the skin, which makes it skin glow
- Smooth fine lines and wrinkles
- Relax the jaw joint (temporomandibular joint or TMJ). Tightness here creates a stress loop increasing anxiety and is linked to the hips.
- Calm the nervous system
- Increase the efficiency of the upper lymph nodes and vessels and help the lower ones too
- Useful for improving sleep, energising, and reducing headaches

Facial acupressure and reflexology techniques stimulate specific points on your face to enhance your overall health and well-being. These techniques can help balance your energy flow, relieve pain and tension, improve lymphatic drainage, and detoxify your skin. They are important influencers of your organs, hormones, emotions, and mood.

Overall, face yoga is a natural and holistic way to improve the health and appearance of your skin, but by including acupressure, reflexology, and deep breathing techniques, takes the effects to a whole new level.

There are visual instructions on my YouTube channel @serenitymojo7134. Head over there and explore the face yoga and breathing videos in the Am I Menopausal playlist.

I will be adding to the content, so subscribe to be notified when there is something new to watch.

Rubbing Points

One of the tools of systematic kinesiology involves rubbing specific points that are based on Chapman reflex points.

Chapman reflex points are small nodules that can be felt under the skin. They are related to the function of different organs and hormone glands in the body. When an organ or gland is not working well, it can cause congestion or a blockage in the lymphatic fluid and affect nerve impulses in the area where the Chapman point is located. This can make the point tender and painful. By rubbing, pressing, or tapping these points, the normal flow of lymph and nerve signals is restored, helping to improve the organ function.

Frederick Mitchell Chapman, an osteopath, found the points based on the connection between the nervous system and the lymphatic system. As already discussed, if we can move the waste via the lymph system it helps the whole body and in particular the organs and hormone glands.

Dr George Goodheart, the founder of Kinesiology, used Chapmans points and found he could link each of them to specific muscles. If a muscle gets injured, becomes tight and tense through physical or emotional stress, or there are changes in your posture, you can rub the related neuro-lymphatic point (rubbing point) to make improvements.

Work all or specific points by rubbing them lightly and quickly. They can feel sharp and painful. Rub for at least 20-30 seconds to feel the reaction. If a point is sore, rub it for up to 1 minute and then return to treat it the following day. Keep treating daily until you have no reaction.

Like any detoxifying treatment you can feel tired, dehydrated, or visit the toilet more often for 24-48 hours after you have rubbed them. This is normal. You may feel euphoric and energised. This is normal too.

Any reaction of a headache, extreme tiredness, feeling more emotional, dizziness, nausea or feeling flu-like, wait until you feel better before rubbing the points again, rest and keep drinking plenty of water.

Use these points when:

- you are emotional or physical stress levels are high
- you have a muscular or skeletal injury, stiffness, or pain
- your hormones are fluctuating
- your emotions are fluctuating
- you are carrying more weight than normal
- you have identified issues with all the areas covered in the chapters in this book including digestion, lymph system, liver
- you sit most of the day

This is not a full list, so locate and rub the points and see how they feel, or you can wake them up by tapping on them all as a morning and evening routine.

Movement

This includes exercise at the gym and sports you may play. For many years now the sport science world have been looking into the effects of fluctuating hormone levels in female athletes. In recent years female athletes have talked about how their monthly cycle affects their ability to train and compete. But what happens when you enter perimenopause?

As you lose oestrogen your type 2 muscle fibres decrease too. These are the fibres that help with activities requiring strength, power, and speed. During the menopause and beyond muscle tone, size, and strength tends to decrease and your muscles take a little longer to recover. On top of this in perimenopause your sleep is often disrupted making you feel fatigue and exhaustion. You may be having hot flushes too and lack motivation.

What Does This all Mean?

If you love your exercise and have been active most of your adult life, think about your body and what it's going through now. Doing the vigorous exercise, at the wrong time of the day, when you are exhausted will trigger a stress response. This means more cortisol being produced and less oestrogen. As discussed previously, symptoms like hot flushes, anxiety, and weight gain especially around the belly will worsen.

What Exercise Should You Do?

It is more important than ever through perimenopause to listen to your body. Your cortisol levels are higher in the morning, and this is the perfect time to exercise and move with vigour. If you are not sleeping well or feel tired when you wake, deal with this first and reduce the intensity of your exercise routine for now.

In the evening, make your exercise routine slower, more stretch orientated, and relaxing by moving all the joints of your body. This will keep your cortisol low and aid your sleep routine by making you feel more comfortable while you sleep.

If you are generally sedentary, find ways to move more throughout the day. You do not need to be at the gym, exercising or playing sport. Choose an activity that you enjoy and incorporate it into your life. This could be walking round the house. You may be trying to drink more water. So set an alarm on your phone every 30 mins to get up to get some water. On the way to fill up your glass you could lung, jog or dance your way there. This may be a little difficult if you are at work in an office with other people but get creative and have fun with it. Encourage others to move with you! An exercise plan should not be a chore. You have earnt the right to enjoy what you do. It may take a while to discover what you like to do, experiment or think back to what you have enjoyed before. I have recently started back taking ballet classes. I enjoyed it when I was a child and now, I am enjoying it again. Ballet is good for the feet, balance, and keeps the brain working too! If you love the gym routine, great! If you need to learn while you exercise, take a class or dance like me. Maybe you love the water or enjoy being part of a team. Working out what you enjoy will keep you active.

If you do not like exercise and shudder at the thought, don't despair look at NEAT (Non-Exercise Activity Thermogenesis). The idea of NEAT comes from the research of James Levine in 2009 and is about getting move movement and activity (not exercise) in everyday life. NEAT is the activity you do and energy you burn while walking to lunch, tapping your toes, folding the washing, and general living. This is for everyone, but especially if you are feeling too tired to exercise, need to lose weight, need to get moving and don't have the motivation. It will help your lymph, decrease your inflammation, give you more energy, and help you improve your health and wellbeing. All you have to do is increase your daily activity. You could stand up when the phone rings and talk while pacing around the room. If your day is filled with meetings, why not walk and talk. Your brain works better when your body is active. Stretch and move your feet when you are sitting in front of the TV or at your desk. Take the stairs or park in a space furthest away from the shop. Washing the car, sweeping leaves, vacuuming all add to your NEAT activity. Every small change to increase in your activity burns more calories, increases your heart rate, and improves your lymphatic system and brain function. Be creative, include your friends and family, and get moving!

For everyone, it is time to focus on strength and stretching. Some women find their muscles and joints become painful and tire easily. Be kind to them and aware of when to stop. Women lose strength as we age. However, before you embark on a weight-training programme get some advice. Be mindful of your energy levels, prioritise your sleep, and concentrate on the health of your lymph, gut, and liver. Deal with these areas first and then make sure you give yourself extra time to recover between sessions.

Keep moving and be active. Listen to your body. Incorporate strength training and gentle stretches. Make sure you do some spinal twists (it will help your breathing, massage your internal organs, and is a movement that most people do not do!). Book in a massage, or reflexology – it is time to start taking care of yourself and these will prevent you from developing injuries that will restrict your movement. Ask the professionals for help and get recommendations for a good physical therapist, massage therapist etc who specialise in working with mid-life clients.

Breathing

Throughout this book you will find specific breathing techniques that help different functions of your body or issues that arise. In truth, all breathing techniques are brilliant if you use them every day. So, pick the one you like and incorporate it into your daily routine. Choose a time or add it on to something you already do each day. Always breath through your nose, that's what it is there for! After just a few days of mouth breathing your stress hormones increase and you crease to filter out the toxins from the air. Nose breathing helps your whole body from fighting infections to calming stress. Most people breathe to much, so once a day slow things down, hold your breath if it comfortable, and train your body to breathe efficiently.

Breathing exercises are easy, and the benefits are huge. Here is what it can do for you:

- Maintain your physical stamina, boosting energy
- Strengthen your voice
- Clarify thinking
- Improve the look, feel and vitality of your complexion
- Energise your eyes
- Relieve tension in the body
- Combat exhaustion and reduce the need for daytime naps
- Assists calmness, peace, and helps to master of your emotions
- Enhances your ability to deal with stress
- Gives your mind and body a break and the time to recover

- Improves the tone of your diaphragm and lung capacity. This in turn gives movement to your abdominal organs providing them with a gentle massage. This helps the lymph system remove waste in the area and brings fresh nutrients in to nourish tissues. Great for the health and function of your digestion and urinary organs.
- Removing more waste and improving the lymph system also gives a boost to your immune system too.

There are visual instructions on my YouTube channel @serenitymojo7134. Head over there and explore the face yoga and breathing videos in the Am I Menopausal playlist

Meditation and Mindfulness

There are many apps and downloadable help to take you through a meditation session accessed from your phone. I always think it is all about the voice and/or music you prefer. Again, to be effective you are better with a few minutes every day than 30 minutes once a week. Regularity of the practice is key.

Bach Flower Remedies

Wonderful subtle remedies that change your emotional and energetic worlds which can influence your physical symptoms too. Each of the 38 remedies can be put into 7 different categories and are for treating a range of personalities and emotions. Taking them is easy. You can put a few drops into your glass of water or directly under your tongue. You can read about these remedies on many good websites and books or by doing a course to learn more about them.

Here is a quick checklist to which ones may suit you and keep checking as your outlook will change over time.

- **Agrimony** – when you are hiding your feelings behind a façade of cheerfulness, dislike arguments and often give in to avoid conflict, and tend to turn to food, alcohol, drugs etc when down
- **Aspen** – if you feel anxious without knowing why, have a secret fear that something bad will happen, and wake up feeling anxious
- **Beech** – you get annoyed by the habits of others, focus on others' mistakes, and are critical and intolerant
- **Centaury** – if you often neglect your own needs to please, find it difficult to say 'no' or are easily influenced
- **Cerato** – when you constantly second-guess yourself, seek advice, and mistrust your own intuition, and change your mind out of confusion
- **Cherry Plum** – you feel afraid I might lose control of myself, have sudden fits of rage, and feel like you are going crazy
- **Chestnut Bud** – you keep making the same mistakes over and over, not learning from experience, and

keep repeating the same patterns

- **Chicory** –you need to be needed and want loved ones close, feel unloved and unappreciated by your family, and are easily slighted and hurt
- **Clematis** – you often feel spacey or absent minded, unable to concentrate for long, and get drowsy and sleep more than necessary
- **Crab Apple** – you seem overly concerned with cleanliness, feel unclean or physically unattractive, and tend to obsess over little things
- **Elm** – you feel overwhelmed by responsibilities, not coping well under pressure, and have temporarily lost your self-confidence
- **Gentian** – you become discouraged with small setbacks, easily disheartened and often sceptical and pessimistic
- **Gorse** – when you feel hopeless and can't see a way out, lack faith that things could get better, and feel sullen and depressed
- **Heather** – when you are obsessed with your troubles, dislike being alone and usually bring conversations back to yourself
- **Holly** – you are suspicious of others, feel discontented and unhappy, full of jealousy, mistrust, or hate

- **Honeysuckle** – you often long for the way things were, think more about the past than the present, and often think about what might have been
- **Hornbeam** – you feel too tired to face the day ahead, mentally exhausted, and tend to put things off
- **Impatiens** – you find it hard to wait for things, are impatient and irritable, and prefer to work alone
- **Larch** – you lack self-confidence, feel inferior becoming discouraged, and never expect anything but failure
- **Mimulus** – if you are afraid of things like spiders, illness etc, are shy, overly sensitive, modest, and get nervous and embarrassed
- **Mustard** – when you get depressed without reason, feel your mood swinging back and forth, and gloomy
- **Oak** – it you tend to overwork and keep going spite of exhaustion, have a strong sense of duty and never give up, and neglect your needs to complete a task
- **Olive** – you feel completely exhausted, physically and/or mentally, totally drained of all energy with no reserves, having been through a long period of illness or stress
- **Pine** – when you feel unworthy, inferior, and guilty, and blame yourself for everything that goes wrong

- **Red Chestnut** – you are overly concerned and worried about loved ones, distressed, and disturbed by other's problems, and worry that harm may come to them

- **Rock Rose** – when you sometimes feel terror and panic, become helpless and frozen with fear, and suffer from nightmares

- **Rock Water** – you set high standards for yourself, are strict with health, work, and/or spiritual discipline, and very self-disciplined, always striving for perfection

- **Scleranthus** – when you find it difficult to make decisions, change your opinion, and have intense mood swings

- **Star of Bethlehem** – if you feel devastated due to recent shock, are withdrawn due to traumatic events, and have never recovered from loss or fright

- **Sweet Chestnut** – you feel extreme mental or emotional heartache, have reached the limits of endurance, and are in complete despair without all hope

- **Vervain** – you get high-strung and very intense, trying to convince others of your way of thinking, and are sensitive to injustice, almost fanatical

- **Vine** – you tend to take charge of projects, situations etc, I consider yourself a natural leader, and are strong-willed, ambitious, and often bossy

- **Walnut** – if you are experiencing change like a move, new job etc, get drained by people or situations, and want to be free to follow ambitions

- **Water Violet** – if you give the impression of being aloof, prefer to be alone when overwhelmed, and often don't connect with people

- **White Chestnut** – you are constantly thinking unwanted thoughts, constantly relive unhappy events or arguments, and are unable to sleep at times because you can't stop thinking

- **Wild Oat** – for when you can't find your path in life, are drifting and lack direction, or you are ambitious but don't know what to do

- **Wild Rose** – feeling apathetic and resigned to whatever happens, with the attitude, 'it doesn't matter anyway', and feel no joy in life

- **Willow** – if you feel resentful and bitter, find it difficult to forgive and forget, and think life is unfair with a 'poor me' attitude

Supplements

During perimenopause, the hormonal changes during this transitional phase can have various effects on your body, and supplements can help address some of these concerns. However, there are important factors you need to consider before introducing supplements into your daily schedule.

All supplements are supplemental to a good healthy diet. There are times when your body needs a little help. This could be when your body is stressed, your digestion or immune systems are compromised, or your body cannot convert the nutrients in the food you feed it into the chemicals required to be of benefit and keep you going. Here using certain supplements may help short-term.

Before taking any supplements, it's crucial to consider your health at the time and consult with a healthcare professional if you are on medication. A systematic kinesiologist or qualified nutritionist can also help you to personalise your choices based on your specific needs, symptoms, and medical history. Additionally, you should prioritise supplements from reputable brands that undergo third-party testing for quality and safety.

It's also important to remember that everyone's experience is unique, and what works for one person may not work for another. For example, most mineral supplements are stabilised with another ingredient attached, like calcium may have carbonate, citrate, malate, or a combination added. It may be a liquid type in the form of calcium chloride. One type may work well with your body and not suit another person. Listen to your body, be aware of any adverse effects or concerns that may arise and take advice.

Nutrient work together for example vitamin D helps the absorption of Calcium and Vitamin K (most of which you get from your gut bacteria) helps to put the calcium in the right place, your bones, and teeth. Taking some supplements long-term can create an imbalance of another nutrient as many work in pairs, like too much zinc can create a copper deficiency. Your body is clever though and will often dump what is does not need via urine. So, taking supplements you do not need can end up as expensive urine and may put extra stress on your liver and kidneys. Having said that Vitamin D with K2 is always a good supplement to take if you are on oestrogen HRT and also for everyone in the winter.

One supplement that is beneficial is omega-3 fatty acids. These fatty acids have anti-inflammatory properties and can potentially alleviate symptoms such as joint pain, mood changes, and cardiovascular concerns during peri-menopause. Remember, before incorporating omega-3 supplementation into your routine, consult with your healthcare professional. This is particularly important if you have any underlying medical conditions, take blood-thinning medications, or other medication as they may interact with the supplement.

B vitamins levels fluctuate with our hormones and are useful if you are feeling anxious, not sleeping, or waking up feeling desperate. I would recommend taking a b complex as they all B's work together. Remember to consult your healthcare professional is you are on medication or your kinesiologist/nutritionist if you want to see if there is a specific B that may need topping up.

Other nutrients to think about are the Marvellous Magnesium which is involved in many processes in the body. Magnesium helps with twitchy legs, heart health, digestive balance, fatigue, insomnia, anxiety, and so much more! Along with Zinc it is the gatekeeper inside every cell in your body. My best advice for ensuring enough magnesium in your body is with Epsom salt baths (I should have shares in Epsom salts!). These salts are full of magnesium and your body will absorb what is needs and leave the rest. Always put at least 1/3 of a kilo in a normal sized bath and relax for 10-20 minutes.

Herbal Supplements

Before considering any herbal supplement, you should consult with a healthcare professional to ensure its safety and discuss potential interactions with any medications you may be taking. Many herbal supplements can be effective, but it is important to get the right one. It is reported that some taken long-term can affect the kidneys or liver. So, it is a good idea to vary them or take a pause every month and as with essential oils. Always buy from the best source, rather than the best price.

Here are some herbal preparations that some women have found helpful for managing menopausal symptoms.

Black cohosh, thought to be helpful for hot flushes, sleep, and mood swings. While the effectiveness of black cohosh is still debated, some individuals find it useful. Keep to the recommended dose and avoid if you have a liver condition.

Red clover, useful for treating hot flushes and the skin dryness, including vaginal. I found this useful at times when I lost confidence and felt a little flat. I would take it for a few days and stop. Some say red clover helps with libido, fatigue and due to its isoflavones content it has the potential to be helpful as you age. With some women in perimenopause found their periods returned. Check with an herbalist if you have had hormone-responsive breast or endometrial cancer.

Ginkgo biloba is used to support cognitive function by increasing the circulation around the brain bringing nourishment and oxygen to your brain cells.

Ashwagandha Root, Siberian and Asian Ginseng, are all effective adaptogens that are great for their calming effect and reducing stress levels. Use them for anxiety, sleep conditions, to protect the ends of your Genes (telomers) that speed up ageing. Do not use if you are prone to intestinal ulcers and check if you have an auto-immune disease.

Turmeric, (and black pepper) is a powerful anti-inflammatory with benefits to the body, brain, and joint health.

Agnus Castus (Chasteberry) has been shown in some studies to influence hormone balance and reduce the severity of some symptoms. Women have reported improvements to sleep and mood. In some cases periods have return which may affect your decision to use this herb.

For more information on herbal preparations and especially if you need further information find and contact an herbalist.

10

HRT

To use or not to use, that is the question!

In the UK oestrogen and progesterone are readily prescribed, but testosterone is not licenced for prescription via the NHS. This may change in the future. Women can be given it to improve sex drive by a specialised doctor. It is given as a gel and rubbed onto the skin. Side effects include unwanted hair growth and acne.

Those who have had a hysterectomy where the uterus has been removed are prescribed oestrogen only. Progesterone is given to protect the lining of the womb and in this case is not necessary.

Types of Oestrogen HRT

Bioidentical hormones are a natural mix of compounds that are tailored to an individual woman's saliva or blood test. These are not supported by NICE in UK (National Institute for Health and Care Excellence). This is due to a lack of consistency in the quality and in some cases the binding agents used, which may be harmful. DHEA is compound made from cholesterol in the body and turned into a oestrogen, progesterone and testosterone. Bioidentical HRT products may use DHEA to increase hormone levels or the specific hormone. However, your body will choose what it makes from the DHEA and this may not be the hormone you want. Products containing progesterone may not be enough to protect the uterus lining.

Body identical HRT are plant-based hormones produced from yams. Most women find they can tolerate these better than synthetic HRT as the chemical structure of these hormones are exactly the same as those your ovaries produce. This means the body recognises it and deals with it much better.

Conjugated oestrogen hormones are an older version of HRT. This form of product comes from pregnant mare's urine and have the best evidence for breast safety when taken on its own. The safety depends on the quality of binders used in production.

Synthetic Oestrogen is never taken orally as it goes through the gut and processed by the liver. Here clotting factors are activated giving an increased risk of DVTs. It also raises blood pressure when it activates the kidneys. Oestrogen from your ovaries is released directly in to the blood and does not go through the digestion like food. Therefore this form of oestrogen is always given through the skin.

Types of Progesterone HRT

Micronized is the natural form of progesterone which is recognised by the body making risks lower. This type of progesterone is not absorbed through the skin as the molecules are too large. It is therefore given in tablet form. As progesterone is a calming hormone with better sleep as a side effect, it is usually suggested to be taken at night.

Synthetic progesterone is also taken by mouth and its effects may differ from naturally produced version from your ovaries. Some types have a growth effect on breast tissue.

Merino Coil device with slow releasing progesterone is an option. The main aim of having progesterone HRT is to protect the womb so this product can be very effective.

Making Your Own Choice

Women under 40 going through menopause are advised to take HRT. For all women, make sure you ask your doctor plenty of questions and make your decision from an informed and personal stand point.

NICE say the prime time to start HRT is in perimenopause, within 10 years of menopause or under 60 years old. This is to receive the optimal benefits. Risks and benefits are individual. So before going to see a professional think about your reason for taking HRT. Is it for the prevention of long-term health benefits, to alleviate symptoms, or both? Most women's symptoms have completely stopped by 60 or before. 1 in 5 have symptoms for the rest of their lives. Taking HRT over 60 may help to alleviate symptoms but will not have the long-term health benefits.

When taking HRT through the skin, the amount that entre your blood stream will differ from person to person. Unlike a tablet where the dose is predictable. The absorption rate of your skin is different to others. This means that if say you and your friend are both on 25mg. Your friend may absorb 20mg while you may only absorb 10mg. After 3 months of starting HRT it is important to have a blood test and follow up appointment to check the levels of oestrogen, progesterone, and testosterone. 50% of testosterone is produced from the ovaries and 50% from the adrenals. The blood test will show whether you have enough testosterone circulating.

If you are on HRT insist on yearly check ups. If you are not taking it a general check up may be a good thing too.

Talking to Your Doctor

Find a doctor in your practice who understands and has had training on menopause. They will be more informed and ready to listen. Take with you information from a symptom tracker, NICE guidance, the British Menopause Society, or your country's equivalent.

Remember to list down you medications, supplements, or herbal remedies and a list of questions or concerns too. This information is also useful when you go to a complementary practitioner. If worried about seeing the doctor, take a friend or family member with you.

What Now?

By now, having read this book, you have a better understanding of what to expect. If you already have some symptoms you may have introduced a few of the tools and are feeling a little better or at least empowered to take control. Once you are calmer and able to cope better it is time to start thinking about what you will do after the menopause and put some plans in place.

It is helpful to see the bigger picture. Post menopause is after all at least a third of your life. So, how are you going to spend it? What will your life to look like? In one of your breathing or relaxing session ask yourself the following questions. You may like to record your answers, work with a buddy, or write down your vision. Have fun, be inspiring, and realistic.

Imagine you are post menopause and living your best life and as healthy as possible:

What does your life look like? Visualise where you are and what you are doing

What do you value most in your vision?

What are you doing more of in your vision?

What are you doing less of in your vision?

What are the key aspects of your vision?

Why is this vision important to you?

When have you experienced aspects of your vision before?

Once you have answers to the above, you could take a picture or produce a mood board to represent your vision. This will be a great way of remembering it. What strengths can you draw upon to achieve your vision and how will you get there?

Menopause is often a time in a woman's life to reconnect with themselves. If you have been a career girl, run a business, family or been the rock for those around you. Now is the time to discover new exciting adventures, or rekindle those you enjoyed in the past. Having a vision of what you would like your life to look like in the future will keep you focused on the destination. It will begin to encourage you to start your journey towards it. Having a vision on the fridge or wall in the bathroom is also for those difficult days, when you need to remember there is still life to be had!

If you are struggling, remember to reach out for help. This could be speaking to a trusted positive friend, counsellor, coach, your hairdresser, or complementary therapist!

Remember, perimenopause is a time of transition. Make it your pivot point and plan the rest of you life now with more dedicated time for yourself.

Interesting Reading

When researching for this book I have used knowledge gained over the last 40 years of practising and never ending training. As a therapist you never know it all! New information is discovered all the time. I have favourite books and website that I use for valuable information.

Here are a few of my favourites:

Books

The Biology of Belief by Bruce H. Lipton, Ph.D.

Why We Sleep by Dr Matthew Walker

Breath by James Nestor

Aromatherapy by Rosemary Caddy

Essential Oil Safety: A Guide for Health Care Professionals *by Robert Tisserand*

Aromatherapy and reflexology Level 3 student notes by Jo Hayns

Essential Oils by Susan Curtis

The Fragrant Mind by Valerie Ann Worwood

The clever gut diet by Dr Michael Mosley

Healthy Gut, Healthy You by Dr Michael Ruscio

Epigenetics the new biology, functional biochemistry clinical reference guide by Chris Astill-Smith

Systematic Kinesiology practitioner's manual by Brian Butler

Essential Kinesiology Techniques for Muscle Testing Practitioner's by Terry Larder

Danielle Collins Face Yoga Method

Facial Reflexology by Marie-France Muller

The Headspace Guide to Mindful Eating: 10 days to Finding Your Ideal Weight by Andy Puddicombe

Management of the Menopause by British Menopause Society

Healing Yoga by Swami Ambikananda Saraswati

Websites

https://askthedentist.com

https://www.mrjamesnestor.com

https://www.sleepfoundation.org

https://www.sleepfoundation.org/sleep-profile-get-started

https://www.sleepfoundation.org/how-sleep-works/chronotypes

https://www.aromaweb.com/

https://www.swanstudy.org/

https://www.youtube.com/watch?v=JJZ8z_nTCZQ

https://www.hormone.org/your-health-and-hormones/endocrine-disrupting-chemicals-edcs

https://www.diabetes.co.uk/body/oestrogen-and-diabetes.html

https://orthopracticeus.com/ce-articles/lifetime-effects-of-mouth-breathing/

https://www.yourhormones.info/hormones/

https://www.bluezones.com/2011/12/the-secrets-of-the-blue-zones/

https://orthopracticeus.com/ce-articles/lifetime-effects-of-mouth-breathing/

https://www.hormone.org/your-health-and-hormones/endocrine-disrupting-chemicals-edcs

https://www.ewg.org/consumer-guides/dirty-dozen-endocrine-disruptors

www.epsomsalts.co.uk

Studies

https://pubmed.ncbi.nlm.nih.gov/24388214/

https://www.sciencedirect.com/science/article/pii/S0306453013002369

https://pubmed.ncbi.nlm.nih.gov/31456736/

https://www.ncbi.nlm.nih.gov/pmc/articles/PMC6466064/

https://pubmed.ncbi.nlm.nih.gov/31456736/

https://pubmed.ncbi.nlm.nih.gov/22902418/

https://pubmed.ncbi.nlm.nih.gov/24388214/

https://pubmed.ncbi.nlm.nih.gov/28303750/

https://pubmed.ncbi.nlm.nih.gov/22475949/

https://www.mdpi.com/2077-0472/5/2/170

https://www.nccih.nih.gov/health/antioxidants-in-depth#:~:text=Antioxidants%20are%20man%2Dmade%20or,be%20beneficial%20in%20preventing%20diseases.

https://pubmed.ncbi.nlm.nih.gov/30057039/

https://www.sciencedirect.com/science/article/abs/pii/S1744388118301750

https://pubmed.ncbi.nlm.nih.gov/31780002/

https://www.sciencedirect.com/science/article/pii/S1877042811029788

About the Author

Jo Hayns has had a 40 year career as a complementary therapist. She has helped and taught many women going through health challenges (and hormone chaos) with holistic lifestyle solutions. Jo believes we can all help ourselves when it comes to living life. She loves to learn, is curious, open-minded, and is always searching for answers.

Her biggest gift is to listen calmly and help her clients make sense of their body in order to find their own solutions. No one size fits all here!

facebook.com/KeepCalmatSerenity

instagram.com/KeepCalmatSerenity

youtube.com/@serenitymojo7134

Printed in Great Britain
by Amazon

35900464R00106